DRAB
to *fab*

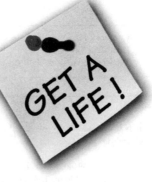

GET A LIFE!

DRAB
to *fab*

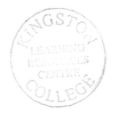

Isabelle Perrett
and
Yvonne Johnson

Hodder Arnold

A MEMBER OF THE HODDER HEADLINE GROUP

Cover © Comstock Images/Getty Images
Hugh Threlfall/Alamy
Donna Day/Stone/Getty Images

Illustrations by Barking Dog Art

The authors would also like to pay special thanks to Hobbs, Wallis, Figleaves, Pirate Verte, Francesco Group, Blissfulbags and Marks and Spencer for kindly providing photographs used in this book.

Photographs   p38, 39, 40, 42, 44, 46, 48 © Photodisc
p50 © Marina Jefferson/The Image Bank/Getty Images
p50 © Adidas 2005
p115 © Royalty-Free/Corbis
p111, 114, 115, 132 © ReproReady.com Limited
p172 © Clark Samuels/Rex Features
p220 © Dennis Wilson/CORBIS

Orders: Please contact Bookpoint Ltd, 130 Milton Park, Abingdon, Oxon OX14 4SB. Telephone: (44) 01235 827720, Fax: (44) 01235 400454. Lines are open from 9.00 to 18.00, Monday to Saturday, with a 24-hour message answering service. You can also order through our website www.hoddereducation.com

British Library Cataloguing in Publication Data
A catalogue record for this title is available from the British Library.

ISBN-10: 0 340 90804 1
ISBN-13: 9 780340 908044

First published   2006
Impression number   10 9 8 7 6 5 4 3 2 1
Year   2008   2007   2006

Copyright © 2006 Isabelle Perrett and Yvonne Johnson

Typeset by Pantek Arts Ltd, Maidstone, Kent.
Printed in Great Britain for Hodder Arnold, a division of Hodder Headline, 338 Euston Road, London, NW1 3BH, by Bath Press, Bath.

Hodder Headline's policy is to use papers that are natural, renewable and recyclable products and made from wood grown in sustainable forests. The logging and manufacturing processes are expected to conform to the environmental regulations of the country of origin.

Every effort has been made to trace copyright for material used in this book. The authors and publishers would be happy to make arrangements with any holder of copyright whom it has not been possible to trace sucessfully by the time of going to press.

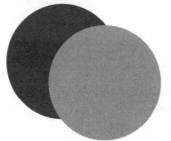

CONTENTS

CONTENTS

CONTENTS

DEDICATION

Isabelle says: The seeds of this book were sown when I was very young by my vivacious and talented French grandmother, whose fabulous creations would arrive through the post in enticing brown paper packages. She inspired in me my passion for image and fashion. I'd like to say thank you to my mother, for being an icon of personal style in her own right, and to both my parents for nurturing in me the belief that we can achieve our dreams with a little effort, and good humour.

Yvonne says: To all my family, friends and clients for your ongoing enthusiasm and support, particularly Carsten and Heather who have played such an important part, often as 'willing' models. Also for my mother; without her influence and enthusiasm I would not have developed such an insatiable love of shopping and clothes.

We'd both like to thank all our friends and clients for their endless patience and constructive comments as we put together the activities in this book. Thanks also to Julia and Paul from First Impressions training for setting us on the practical path of helping our clients look good, feel great and turn heads.

INTRODUCTION

Welcome to *Drab to Fab*, the book that will transform your looks, confidence and self-esteem. Whether you're a teenager or a new mum, a career woman or home-maker, you deserve to look good and feel special about yourself.

Allow us to introduce ourselves – we are Isabelle Perrett and Yvonne Johnson, two trained image consultants and coaches with a passion for developing people. Whether at home or at work, we help people like you grow from the inside out. We have witnessed first hand the power that a positive mental attitude has in helping you achieve your dreams.

This book focuses on personal image – how to make the most of your looks. But most importantly, it focuses on how you feel about your looks. We live in a society that defines people by their appearance. We believe that's unhealthy and leads us to constantly compare ourselves against unrealistic and unattainable icons. Did you know that models in magazines are mostly airbrushed? Or that if shop mannequins were real women they'd be too thin to menstruate?

As two working mothers, we know it's impossible to look your best every minute of every day – and we wouldn't want to, even if we could! Living a life that involves being dolled to the nines at all hours of day and night, is a recipe for stress and distress. What's important is to live life to the full, to accept your body as it is now, and to know how to turn on the style when it counts. We rejoice that women come in all shapes and sizes. We want you to emphasise your assets rather than fret about your figure flaws.

By sharing with you the secrets of style success, our mission is to help you be comfortable in your own skin, to make the most of what you have and who you are now, and to know how to make a positive impression when you need to.

So how can this book help? For a start, it's designed as a programme with each step building on the last. Like shifting your weight or learning to drive, making lasting changes to your image involves changing habits – one step at a time.

Because you are unique, the first chapter includes a self-diagnosis tool to help you identify the specific areas that are important for you. That means you can either follow the steps as building blocks, or you can focus on the bits you need and leave out those you don't. To help you on your way, there's also an optional extra – a daily text message to remind and encourage you as you make progress.

This book covers all aspects of personal presentation – not just your clothes and beauty routine. There are sections on self-image, posture and body language, interviews and socialising. We've included advice on looks for different personalities, situations and lifestyles. Understanding what suits your body shape and colouring is one thing, but it's got to work for your age, mood and budget too. All these will help you to stand out from the crowd and get noticed for the right reasons.

Above all, this book will help you be yourself and have fun doing it. Our promise to you is that in 100 days (you can speed up or slow down the programme as you wish), you can transform forever the way you see yourself and the way others see you. So say goodbye to Drab and hello to Fab!

Isabelle Perrett and Yvonne Johnson

Daily Text Message Service

 A unique, interactive text messaging service is available★ with this book. Daily texts provide inspiration as well as key tips and advice to help you achieve your goal.

By subscribing at the beginning of a 10-day period you will receive a message each day encouraging you and supporting the guidance already given in the book for that day.

So, what are you waiting for? Text the keyword on Day 1 to 80881 to receive invaluable advice that will help you to achieve your full transformation.

★ UK only

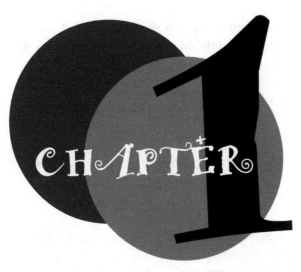

CHAPTER 1

WHO ARE YOU?

Subscribe now to your set of 10 daily text messages. Just text 'Fab 1' to 80881 and receive the advice and encouragement you need to go from *Drab* to *Fab*.

Each set of messages costs £1.50. Please see page xiii for full terms and conditions.

100 days to a new you

This book is for women who think they're drab and want to be fab.

This book will change forever the way you see yourself and the way others see you. You will grow in confidence and your self-esteem will blossom. And all this without needing a surgeon's nip'n'tuck.

> 'The secret of getting ahead is getting started.' Mark Twain, American writer

This book offers a step-by-step programme to a new you. With so much information already available, how can this book help?

- Big changes happen in small steps – instant makeovers are for fashion shoots, not real life. This programme will transform you in 100 days – but of course, feel free to speed up or slow down according to your needs. However fast you progress, prepare to be amazed.
- You have to put it into practice. It's one thing to read style advice in a magazine – it's another to try out new ideas for real. With each daily activity, you'll take a tangible step towards the goal of a new you.
- Change from the inside out. Developing a great image isn't just about what you wear – it's about developing a positive state of mind. In this book, the activities are designed to work on your inner thoughts as well as your outer image.
- Advice from experts. Every piece of advice and every activity has been road tested on hundreds of happy clients. There's no room here for screaming fashion tips that will be dated by the time you've finished the book.
- Above all, it's about discovering who you are and having fun – whether you're doing this on your own or with friends.

Activity

Get armed, get ready

- Gather as much information as you can. The more inspired you are, the more you'll learn. Here are just a few of our favourites. Can you add to the list?

  - Books:
    What Your Clothes Say About You, Trinny Woodall and Susannah Constantine
    The Body Image Workbook, Thomas F. Cash
    Instyle: Secrets of Style, Lisa Arbetter
    Body Talk, Judi James
    Coach Yourself to Feel Great, Amanda Lowe
  - Magazines:
    InStyle
    Eve
    Marie Claire
    Hello
    OK
  - Internet:
    Check out sites like
    net-a-porter.com
    handbag.com
    uniquelywoman.co.uk

- Take a look in the TV listings. What are the current makeover programmes? Can you video them to pick up some tips?

- Keep all of these sources of information and inspiration to hand throughout the programme. You will need them for some of the activities.

WHO ARE YOU?

3

Do you need help?

Your image matters. It has a huge impact on others and also affects how you feel about yourself. We all know the feeling of a 'bad hair day'.

This chapter explores the nature of your image and what it means. You'll look at and challenge your values and beliefs – who is the real you? How do your inner thoughts affect you on the outside? You'll see how your ideal image helps you to feel happier about yourself.

TOP TIP

♦ Buy yourself a notebook to jot down your thoughts and personal notes – it'll help you see how much progress you're making.

What's image anyway?

Your image is an important part of how you communicate. It's made up of lots of components – your appearance, how you use your body, words to express how you feel, even your charisma. Your image can be compared to your own personal packaging; the way others see you. What is the first impression you create?

A positive image isn't about 'beauty or the beast'. You will learn how to let the real, attractive you shine through, whatever your shape, age or colouring. Remember, the most important thing you can step out with isn't a Prada bag or a pair of Earl jeans, but a positive frame of mind.

WHO ARE YOU?

Activity

Let's get quizzical...

Answer 'yes' or 'no' to the following:

1. Do you know what makes you unique and different?

2. Would others say you radiate confidence?

3. Do you buy items to update your look?

4. Do you know how to flatter yourself by choosing the right colours and styles?

5. Do you regularly wear most of what's in your wardrobe?

6. When meeting others for the first time do you generally get a positive reaction?

7. Is clothes shopping enjoyable?

8. Does your make-up look good?

9. Can you list at least five positive things about your image?

10. Can you decide quickly which clothes to wear for most occasions?

How did you do? Score 1 point for each 'yes' and 0 for 'no'.

4 or less This book will really help you.

5–8 Select your areas of focus – go for it.

8 or more Great, let's improve on perfection.

WHO ARE YOU?

5

Go for your goals

As you work through this book you will read about important things which you may want to change about yourself or your image. Your desire to change is a good start – this book is about making it happen. How many times have you thought about making a change, but never actually done anything about it?

⊚✎ TOP TIP

- Always break a massive goal into smaller steps. You'll feel positive and motivated if you can celebrate your successes along the way. It's like eating a six-course meal – all on one plate, it would be too much!
- To help you along your journey you can subscribe to a daily text message as a reminder.

Go for it

To make something happen you must be clear what your goal is and have the drive to see it through. Half-hearted hopes won't get you your dreams.

'If at first you don't succeed, try and try again.' Anonymous

Activity

The massive goal principal

Think of a pyramid – massive and awe-inspiring – what an achievement! You can do this with your own goals.

- Think about what your really important image-related goal is – it can be as big as you like. The bigger the better.

- Draw a pyramid on a large piece of paper. Each block represents one step towards your goal.

- Think of things you will have to do to achieve the goal and list them in order of importance. Write each mini goal in a block with the most important tasks at the bottom of the pyramid. Ensure each block is specific and achievable. (For example, 'I will buy underwear which makes me feel sexy.')

- Keep focused on the large goal, but as you complete each mini goal, cross it out on your pyramid.

- Don't be afraid to add to and change your goals as you proceed on your journey.

- Never give up! And always celebrate your achievements.

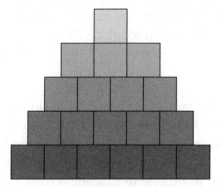

Most important

Source: Adapted from David Hyner, www.stretchdevelopment.co.uk

Goal description

_____
_____
_____
_____
_____
_____
_____
_____

WHO ARE YOU?

Ideal to real

'Those who are going nowhere usually get there.' Henry Ford, founder of the Henry Ford Motor Company

Your mind is incredibly powerful when it comes to achieving what you want in life. Imagine a weight lifter who doubted whether he could lift a certain weight – he wouldn't stand a chance! It's just the same with you. If you tell yourself you'll never look attractive or will never lose weight, you won't. By reinforcing these negative thoughts you reinforce their power.

> **FACT:** Research suggests that increasing positive thinking can extend your lifespan by up to 10 years!

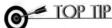 TOP TIP

♦ Find a picture of yourself taken when you were truly happy. Stick it in a place where you'll see it every day – on the fridge, for example. When you look at it, you can recall these positive feelings and focus on them.

However, the good news is that you can use your mind in a positive way, to make a real difference. You can overcome obstacles in your life through reprogramming, changing your subconscious mind with positive beliefs, visions and expectations. If you want something to change for you then you need to be able to imagine it first. See what happens when you try.

WHO ARE YOU?

Activity

Your idol

- Give yourself some space. Sit in an area where you can relax and won't be disturbed.

- Think of someone you really admire. It can be anyone – a famous personality or a friend.

- Jot down the characteristics of this person and the sorts of words or types of things they might say.

- Now imagine them walking into a room. How would they look? How would they act and speak? What would other people's reactions be to them?

- Imagine yourself walking into that same room. Visualise how you would look, act and feel.

- Now repeat the scenario – but this time you're in the skin of your idol.

- Feel that confidence! How do you feel on the inside? What do you look like? How do you express yourself through words and gestures? How do others react to you?

- Does being in someone else's skin create a different outcome for you?

- Practise this for different situations. Use your mind to transform the ideal into the real.

WHO ARE YOU?

Accentuate the positive

Focusing on the positive aspects of your image, however small, is your first step to the new you. To do this you need to take an honest look at yourself.

Many women find it hard to be objective, let alone positive, about their looks. We are bombarded by warped images of beauty, which lead us to focus on our imperfections. Today's activity is about starting to look at yourself realistically, to recognise the positive and to identify a few, selected aspects of your appearance that you'd like to improve.

'There are 3 billion women who don't look like supermodels and only eight who do.' The Body Shop advertising campaign, 1997.
Reproduced with kind permission of The Body Shop International plc.

Activity Take a look at yourself

- Take a deep breath and stand naked, or in your underwear, in front of the mirror. Look at your reflection face on, sideways and over your shoulder at the back view.

- Take a good look at your posture.

- Start at your head and work down. List five things you like about your body and write them down on the chart opposite. Think about what you can do with your body as well as how it looks. You must write at least five things!

- Now do the same for the bad bits. List **no more than** three things.

- Ask yourself what you're already doing to accentuate the positives.

WHO ARE YOU?

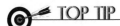 TOP TIP

- Ensure you've got a full length mirror – and don't be afraid to use it.
- If you find it hard to do this activity on your own, ask a friend to help.

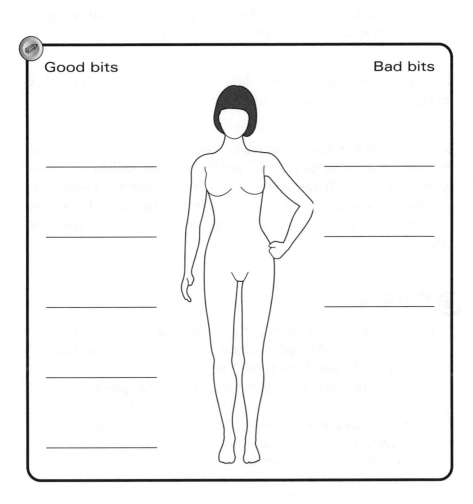

Good bits

Bad bits

_____   _____

_____   _____

_____   _____

_____

_____

WHO ARE YOU?

11

Through someone else's eyes

Working on your image – the way you look and sound, the way you move – requires you not only to be honest with yourself but also to see yourself as others see you.

Some people have a good understanding of the strengths and weaknesses of their own image. They recognise which positive aspects they want to emphasise and which they want to camouflage.

Others, however, find it more difficult to be objective about their image. Do you know how others see you?

Seeing yourself through someone else's eyes isn't always about revealing your blind spots – the muffin-top rolls spilling over your jeans, for example. It can reveal some pleasant surprises. Others may see qualities you didn't know you had, like an infectious laugh. Can you convey a whole range of emotions through your eyes? Have you got great ankles?

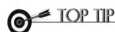 TOP TIP

- ◆ Don't ask your mother or best friend for feedback. They will find it hard to be objective. Ask people who will give you helpful and honest feedback.
- ◆ If you can't find anyone to ask, take a photograph or, better still, a video of yourself from different angles – front, back and side views. When you look at them, answer the questions as though you were seeing yourself through someone else's eyes.

WHO ARE YOU?

Today's activity is about helping you understand the positive and negative aspects of your image so that you can use them to maximum advantage.

Activity

Assess your image

1. Take a photo of yourself as you typically look now and stick it in your notebook.

2. Ask yourself the following questions about your image:

   ● What's the first thing that comes to mind when I think of myself?

   ● What three words would I use to describe my overall image?

   ● What's the best thing about the way I look?

   ● What's the worst thing about the way I look?

   ● How would I describe my voice and way of speaking?

   ● How would I describe my body language and gestures?

   ● What one thing could I do to improve my image?

3. Now ask three people whom you know and trust to answer the same questions about you.

4. Compare their answers with yours. Are there any shocks or surprises? What does it tell you about your image and the way you see yourself?

WHO ARE YOU?

Your mantra

In his book *The Naked Woman*, Desmond Morris explains how the most gorgeous women in the world are those who combine the two qualities of physical and behavioural beauty. That's why in recent surveys Kylie Minogue, Helen Mirren, Catherine Deneuve and Honor Blackman have topped the lists of the sexiest women of their generations.

Not all of these women are conventionally beautiful but they are sexy by virtue of their talent, intelligence and lack of prudery. In their own way, they all exude self-confidence.

'Human beings, by changing the inner attitudes of their minds, can change the outer aspects of their lives.'
William James, American psychologist and philosopher

It's no secret that if you repeat something to yourself often enough you will start to believe that it's true. And if you believe it's true, you'll start to behave differently. In turn, others will start to respond to you in a different way.

Today's activity is about developing a really powerful positive phrase and using it to change your view of yourself. Buddhists call such phrases mantras and have used them for centuries to harness the power of personal belief. Modern psychology uses similar techniques such as neuro linguistic programming (NLP) to help people achieve different results in their lives by changing the way they think.

WHO ARE YOU?

Activity

Define your mantra

- Go over the self-review exercises you have carried out over the last few days. Pick one positive aspect of your image now. Use it to develop a positive mantra like this:

I love my/the way ...

_____

_____

_____

because ...

_____

_____

_____

The positive effect this has on others is ...

_____

_____

_____

- Repeat your mantra at least three times a day for the coming week. Make it part of your routine – you might want to do it each time you brush your teeth.

- When you've done this for a week, make a note of any changes in the way you feel about yourself, and any changes in the reaction you've had from others. What's started to happen?

WHO ARE YOU?

15

All wrapped up

Human beings are like presents – all wrapped up. Only a small fraction of your identity is visible on the surface. Most of who you are and what you stand for is hidden beneath the wrapping. Beauty is only skin deep. Attractiveness is about what lies beneath the surface.

Have you ever stopped to think about what makes you unique and attractive? If not, how can you be sure that the image you project to the outside world is really you? For example, you may be creative, full of ideas, or someone who enjoys being different and standing out from the crowd. Do you dare to show this on the outside, or do you hide the inner you?

A powerful and positive personal image isn't just about looking good – it's about saying who you are and what you stand for. A product has a brand, which is instantly recognisable and conveys what it's about. Similarly, how you look, sound and behave make up your personal brand – who you really are.

Understanding yourself is the starting point to developing confidence and a unique personal style that makes a statement about who you are.

Activity

If you were a present

- Take a blank sheet of A4 paper and fold it in half. Divide it into two columns.

- List up to 10 things about yourself that you'd really like to shine through. These might be personal qualities, skills, experience or things you'd like others to know about you. Here are some examples: 'I am someone who thrives on variety. I can come up with new ideas. I have a good eye for colour when it comes to decorating. I believe in having fun.'

If I were a present

10 things I'd like to shine through:

If I were a present, I'd look like this:

1. _____

2. _____

3. _____

4. _____

5. _____

6. _____

7. _____

8. _____

9. _____

10. _____

● Now use the descriptions of your inner qualities to draw what kind of present you would be. Think about:

  – it's size, shape, weight and the way it's labelled.
  – and finally, what's inside?

● Now compare the results from Day 6. How much of the real you shines through? What changes to your image might you want to make?

WHO ARE YOU?

Your notes

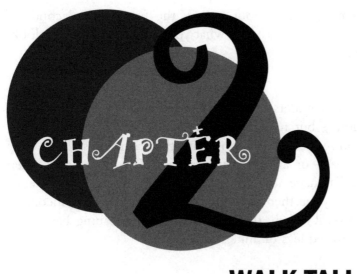

CHAPTER 2

WALK TALL

Body talk

How clearly do you communicate? Your body talks whether you like it or not. You give signals to others about how you feel and who you are through your body language.

First impressions count

People make judgements about you in the first 20–30 seconds of meeting you. This is not based on what you say, but on how you look, move and sound.

Being able to read, understand and use body language is a key skill of communication – but remember that it isn't an exact science. For example, if you see someone sitting with their arms crossed, are they feeling defensive – or are they simply cold? For this reason, when reading body language it is important to look for other evidence which supports your theory. In the example above, if someone is feeling defensive, it's likely that they will also be leaning backwards slightly with crossed legs or ankles too.

> 'Fie, fie upon her!
> There's language in her eye, her cheek, her lip,
> Nay, her foot speaks; her wanton spirits look out
> At every joint and motive of her body.'
> William Shakespeare, Trolius and Cressida, IV, 5

WALK TALL

Liar, liar, pants on fire ...

Your body language doesn't lie. In fact, this tendency makes it hard for anyone to lie convincingly using words as your gestures and actions will often give you away. Think about small children – their actions definitely speak louder than words as delight, sadness, anger and fury are easy to see and read.

Activity **Read the signs**

- Watch your favourite reality TV programme, such as *Big Brother*.

- Turn the sound down and notice people – their gestures, their arms, hands, face, eyes, head and posture.

- Can you identify the emotions they appear to be going through?

- Now turn the sound up and see if you were right. Notice how the body language changes depending upon how uptight, happy, angry or sad each person is feeling.

FACT: Studies show that if your body language matches your words, you're four times more likely to get your message across.

WALK TALL

Perfect posture

If posture is a word that conjures up pictures of young ladies at finishing school walking around with books on their heads, then think again. Posture is vital. It refers not just to how you hold your body, but also how you move it.

Posture has an impact on how others see you. You can use your posture just as much as your gestures and facial expression to express interest and openness.

Consider, for example, a woman with hunched shoulders and her head down shuffling towards you. She greets you with a whispered 'hello' muttered to her shoes. Not exactly a positive impression.

On the other hand, she could walk with an upright stance, her head facing forwards, her shoulders back and her hand outstretched to shake yours. 'Hello!' she beams.

Which woman would make the more positive impression?

Your posture may have become a force of habit, but it also reflects how you feel about yourself, and over time it can affect your health. An arched back, hunched shoulders and drooping head can all contribute to back problems, breathlessness and indigestion due to scrunched organs.

People who stand tall ooze confidence. And the good news is that good posture can help you to appear several pounds lighter as well as help relieve tension in your body. Many back and neck problems are caused by or worsened by slouching or poor posture. A positive posture will get a positive response, and will reinforce those good feelings about yourself.

WALK TALL

Activity

Proper posture

1. Stand in comfortable clothes in a quiet room and take your shoes off. Move your feet a hip-width apart.

2. Starting from your pelvis, zip your tummy muscles in and up towards your chest. Pilates followers will be familiar with this exercise.

3. Shrug your shoulders to help relieve tension, then gently roll your shoulders backwards. When you've done that three times, roll your shoulders forwards.

4. As you do so, make sure you breathe in and out fully. Breathing helps you relax and will encourage a relaxed but upright posture.

5. Now imagine that your neck is lengthening and your head is lifting away from your body. Make sure you keep looking straight ahead.

6. Finally, imagine you're a puppet suspended from an invisible thread going all the way through your body from your pelvis, through your torso and up through the roof of your head.

7. Now walk forward, imagining you're being pulled by that thread. Keep your tummy in, shoulders back and head up.

How different does that feel from your usual walk? Really try to keep it up all day and see how you feel. Notice the positive reactions you get from other people.

WALK TALL

Presenting with panache

Is making a presentation one of your greatest fears? You're not alone. If just thinking about it gives you the jitters – don't panic.

A key part of being successful at presentations is how you come across, particularly in those first few moments. At no time can you afford to get sloppy if you want to impress your audience.

So, how can you make that all-important impression?

DOs

- Rehearse your opening three times until you don't need notes. Concentrate on your body language as well as the words.
- Walk into the room with your head held high. Use your posture to look interested and enthusiastic.
- Accompany your opening remarks with open gestures – perhaps some arm movement to emphasise what you're saying. Maybe a smile?
- Face the audience and project your voice.
- Take your hands out of your pockets. Move them occasionally to illustrate your key points.
- Keep your posture positive – head up, stand tall.
- Scan the audience. What are they saying? Look out for encouraging nods, eye contact or smiles.

DON'Ts

Do not:
- Cross your arms or wave them around uncontrollably.
- Rock backwards and forwards.
- Use the table as a prop.
- Turn your back to the audience.
- Stare at the screen.

WALK TALL

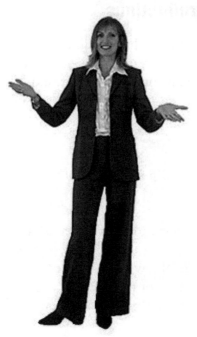

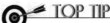

TOP TIP

- Before any presentation spend a few minutes speaking positively to yourself. Tell yourself how great you are and that the audience is really looking forward to meeting you. Don't allow yourself to think that your presentation could be anything other than fantastic.
- Join a public speaking group like Toastmasters International to brush up on your skills.

Activity

Presentation perfection

- Watch a presenter you admire – it can be on TV or live.

- Study how they make an impact. What body language do they use? How do they create rapport with the audience?

- Now practise your presentation using these techniques – preferably capture this on video or watch yourself in the mirror.

- Give yourself loads of feedback – and keep on practising what works.

WALK TALL

Inspiring interviews and introductions

Going for an interview? Meeting someone for the first time? Whether at work or at play, see this as an opportunity to shine – the other person is keen to see you, they are anticipating you'll be great. Body language and appearance are crucial in making that great first impression. Follow the steps below for success.

♦ Do your homework. Find out about the person, the company, the job.
♦ Dress smartly and appropriately.
♦ 'Walk tall'. Slouching or timidly entering a room will create a poor first impression.
♦ Handshake? Keep it firm and positive. No 'wet fish' please.
♦ If it's a job, dress for the job you want – not the one you've got.
♦ Think of reasons why you'd be great for this job, why you really want it.

FACT: One in four job applicants fails because of his or her appearance, according to an online poll of 700 job-seekers and employers.

Source: online survey by fish4jobs, 2002

 TOP TIP

♦ If you're unsure of your handshake, ask for constructive feedback from a friend or colleague.
♦ If you go for an interview, always ask for feedback afterwards.

WALK TALL

The good news is that you can appear confident without saying a word. Confidence is a state of mind and is reflected in the way you look, move and behave – not just in what you say.

Think 'BLESSOR' and you won't go wrong:

Breathe.
Lean forward to show interest.
Eye contact.
Smile.
Sit straight and face the interviewer.
Open body language. No crossed arms/legs.
Relax. No hunched shoulders.

Activity

3... 2... 1... action!

- Ask a friend to give you some practice at interviews or initial introductions – ask for feedback afterwards.

- Even better, video the experience and look at how you come across. Jot down your strengths and any areas to improve upon.

WALK TALL

Crafty confidence

Dressing up is a great way to explore aspects of your personality that don't usually shine through. How many of us wish we could be more assertive, confident, adventurous, impulsive, organised, dramatic…? Well, today you'll have your chance.

In her recent TV programme, *A Week of Dressing Dangerously*, presenter Angela Buttolph encouraged participants to bring out the hidden sides of their character and change how they felt, simply by choosing different clothes.

Children are great at this. Today is your chance to have a go at revealing the hidden you.

For example, if you want to bring out your powerful side, perhaps you could pick more structured clothes in blocks of colour. Stick to plain, dark fabrics with sharp, crips lines – possibly a suit. Avoid frills and flowery patterns. Wear polished make-up and tie your hair back or wear it in a sleek, smooth style. Choose simple but stylish jewels – perhaps something metal. Finish it off with high black heels to add height, and a designer bag.

At first, this activity is bound to feel a little strange, but stick with it. As you relax into your alter ego, you will see how you approach situations differently, and how other people respond differently to you.

Activity

Try on a new personality

1. Pick one aspect of your personality that doesn't usually shine through – one you'd like to emphasise. Write down in your notebook some ideas about that quality.

2. Now ask a friend to put together a 'look' that you can wear for a day. Let them rummage through your wardrobe and perhaps through their own to seek inspiration. If you've got children, perhaps it's time to raid their dressing-up box. Failing everything, get down to the local charity shop. If you have some ideas of your own, why not contribute them too?

3. Now the challenge is to wear the look for a day and go about your normal activities, but emphasising all the time the hidden quality you want to shine through. Try to behave as though this really is perfectly normal.

4. How does it make you feel? What reaction do you get from others? What's positive about your experience? What didn't you enjoy?

WALK TALL

Trust me

Creating trust is important whether you're in a social or a business situation. Maybe you're trying to convince someone to buy your products, perhaps you fancy that special person or maybe you're building a great new friendship. If things are going to progress further the other person needs to trust you. Using the right body language will help you to build this trust – although remember it's not always a quick process. Don't get full-on because you assume you've built trust after only two minutes.

Personal space

First, watch you don't get too close. We all have our own personal space which surrounds us. Close-to (around 30-60 cm) is only for your nearest and dearest; from 60 cm is good once someone knows you; and a body's width apart is best for someone you've just met. Be aware that if someone keeps backing off, it's probably not your perfume. It's more likely that you may be standing a little close.

In the UK we tend to have bigger personal space zones than other countries. Be aware of this if you travel or meet someone of a different nationality.

FACT: Road rage often starts because someone has invaded the space around our car – we like to 'own' this space and hate it being invaded by someone driving too close or stealing 'our' parking space.

WALK TALL

Mirroring

When you're talking to someone, try to mirror how they talk – their tone, speed and volume. Mirroring their body language – the way they're sitting or standing, their use of hands and arms – can also be very powerful.

Take care not to be too obvious. You will notice when you watch people who are in rapport with each other that these things happen without them even thinking about it.

Activity

Smile please!

- For a day, practise smiling more. Smile at people you wouldn't normally smile at.

- What response do you get?

- How does it make you feel?

Like a magnet

Have you ever tried to convey your interest in someone and failed because you lack confidence? Maybe you've looked on enviously as someone else fills the room with their presence and leaves you in the corner like a shrinking violet. Remember though, you can convey your interest and appear confident without even saying a word. Confidence is a state of mind and the way you look and act will contribute hugely to how confident you feel.

One thing you can do is to make sure you feel great in what you're wearing, as this will impact directly on your feelings about yourself. If you step into a room feeling like a million dollars, this will show in everything you say and do. People will notice you and maybe compliment you, you'll then feel even better about yourself. With this boost to your self-esteem there'll be no stopping you!

On top of the message you send out through the clothes you wear, of course other non-verbals are really important too. When you're attracted to someone your body language is hard to conceal. Although this may happen unconsciously, it's worthwhile being aware of the signals you can send to show you're interested.

Typical ways for a woman to show she is interested:

- ◆ Lean forwards, nod and smile.
- ◆ Eye contact is important. The longer you hold your eye contact, and the more frequently you make eye contact, the greater your interest.
- ◆ You may sit with legs twined and pointing towards your object of interest.
- ◆ Feet pointing towards your intended are a sure way to convey interest.
- ◆ If all else fails, your parting shot can be a gentle peck on the cheek!

WALK TALL

And here's how you know he's interested:

◆ 'The gaze' – where his eyes follow you round the room or meet yours frequently. Dilated pupils are a subconscious sign that he's interested too.

◆ He's holding his stomach in and chest out.

◆ Preening. Is he smoothing his hair down, straightening his tie or dusting himself down?

◆ Hands on hips? Torso pointing in your direction? Watch out – he's interested.

Activity
Fancy your chances

● Next time you're out and you see someone you'd like to get to know better, watch out for positive signals from their body language.

● Be bold – make eye contact.

● Perhaps introduce yourself and find out more.

● Practise signalling your interest and see the response.

● Keep practising – it really does get easier.

WALK TALL

Your notes

....

....

....

....

....

....

....

....

....

....

....

....

....

....

....

CHAPTER 3

PLAY WITH COLOUR

Colour conundrum

It's time to start looking at how to make the most of your looks. Wearing the right colours on the right bits of your body can transform you from a bag lady to a super diva. Colour savvy chicks buzz with life, look attractive, slim, healthy, self-assured, coordinated – oh, and younger!

So if colour can do so much, why do so many women shroud themselves in black? Firstly, black is safe – it's chic, it goes with pretty much everything else, and it's slimming. Secondly, too many women don't know what colours suit them and are afraid to experiment. The choice of colours in the shops is confusing and just a little scary.

The good news is that anyone can wear any colour – except pure black and white as these two colours, when worn next to the skin, make some people look ill or washed out. It's the quality of colour that counts, and what you wear it with.

First, some colour facts to help you understand what to look for: all colours have three qualities – undertone, clarity and depth.

The **undertone** describes whether it has more blue or yellow in the mix. Blue colours are cool, yellow ones are warm.

The **clarity** describes whether a colour is clear, pure and bright, or soft and dusky, mixed with grey.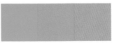

The **depth** of a colour relates to how much black or white is in the mix.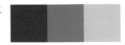

Over the next week or so, you'll learn the qualities of colour that suit you, what to wear them with, and the effect they have on other people.

Activity

The daylight test

- Do this activity in daylight and make sure you use a mirror near a window. It won't work under artificial light. Remove your make-up and pull your hair off your face so you can see your natural colouring.

- Pick out the clothes from your wardrobe and sort them into piles by colour. Never mind whether or not you like them. For example, make a pile of reds, another pile of blues and so on.

- Make a list like this in your notebook:

Colours I look best in	Colours I look worst in	Colours I've never considered

- Taking a pile at a time, hold each item to your face. Do people compliment you when you wear it? Does it bring out your eye colour? Does it give you a healthy glow and lift your face, or do you look ill and tired? Does it give you a clear skin or show every pimple and crease? If it's flattering, keep it. If not, ditch it.

- Now you should have much smaller piles with colours and shades that really work for you. The next few days will help you understand why some shades work for you and others don't.

PLAY WITH COLOUR

Mirror, mirror

Understanding which colours really suit you depends on your natural colouring. It's amazing how many people don't actually know the precise colour of their eyes. Do you?

Today's activity helps you get to grips with the real you – here and now. If you find this activity hard, do it with a friend.

You will use the results of your observation over the next few days to work out which colours suit you best, and why.

Activity Know your colouring

- In natural daylight, look at your eyes in the mirror and tick which is most like you:

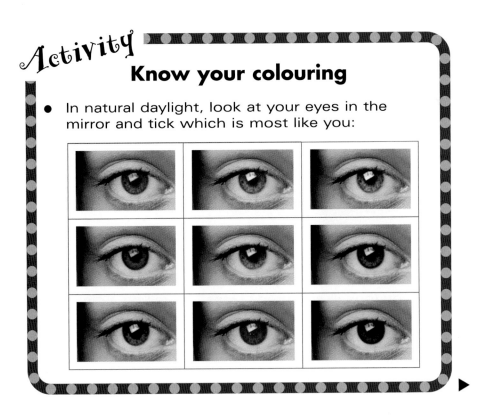

● Now look at your skin. How would you describe it? Choose one from each row.

Pale	Medium	Deep
Warm – olive, golden, freckled, golden brown	Neutral – beige, neither warm nor cool	Cool – rosy, pinkish, bluish, sallow

● And what about your hair? If your hair is dyed, work with the dyed colour, or the colour you are aiming for when you next apply colour to your hair.

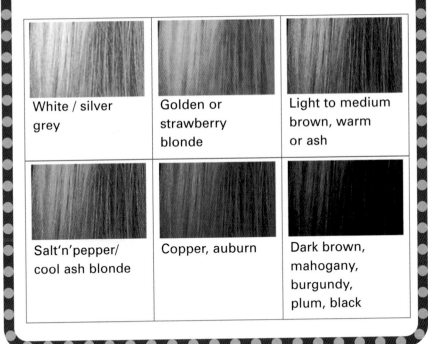

White / silver grey	Golden or strawberry blonde	Light to medium brown, warm or ash
Salt'n'pepper/ cool ash blonde	Copper, auburn	Dark brown, mahogany, burgundy, plum, black

PLAY WITH COLOUR

Is your undertone warm?

The best colour in the world is the one that looks good on you. The key to wearing colours with confidence is knowing what will flatter the colour of your skin, eyes and hair. Let's start by looking at whether you're best suited to golden, warm tones. So many women get this wrong and it can result in

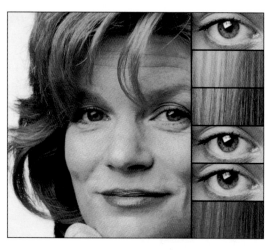

hideous mistakes – hair that heaves, lipstick that screams and foundation that makes you look ill.

Activity

Are you a golden girl?

- Working in daylight and without make-up, hold a piece of white paper to your face. This will really show the undertone of your skin. If your skin looks warm, golden or creamy, tans easily or has obvious freckles, you have a warm undertone.

- Now look at your eyes and hair and do the same. If your eyes are brown, hazel, dull green or teal blue, and your hair is auburn, ginger, golden brown or blonde, you have a warm undertone.

- Look at your favourite colour piles. Do they match the suggestions opposite? If so, you are a golden girl - check out the guidelines on the opposite page.

- If not, wait until the next step to see if you're an ice maiden.

PLAY WITH COLOUR

Famous golden girls include Nicole Kidman and Sarah Ferguson.

Colours to suit a golden girl

What colours suit you?

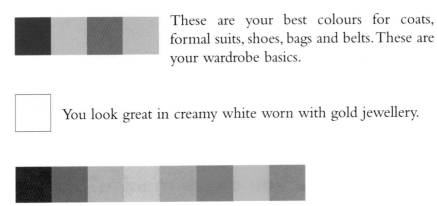

These are your best colours for coats, formal suits, shoes, bags and belts. These are your wardrobe basics.

You look great in creamy white worn with gold jewellery.

These are good colours to mix and match with. Use them for clothes, make-up and accessories.

How should you wear your favourite colours?

Always combine your favourite colours with other colours that have a warm undertone.

Colours that kill

Your worst colours are those with a cool, icy quality. If you can't avoid them, make sure you wear warmer shades next to your face and try to blend cool and warm shades in the same colour – for example, sky blue mixed with a warm turquoise. If you wear white metals, make sure they're matt, rather than shiny.

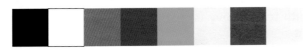

PLAY WITH COLOUR

Is your undertone cool?

If your undertone isn't warm, perhaps you're more suited to shades that have a blue, icy quality about them.

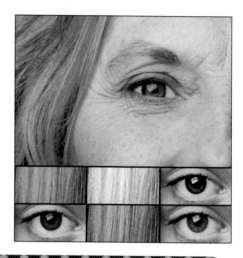

Activity

Are you an ice maiden?

- Working with a mirror in daylight, find some gold wrapping paper and a piece of tin foil and hold these one at a time to your face. What do you notice? If you have a cool undertone, your skin will be rosy, beige or even oriental. The silver foil will enhance your skin tone, giving you a fresh, clear-skinned look. The gold paper will make you look grey and washed out.

- Now look at your eyes and hair. Ice maidens often have eyes that are blue, blue grey or greyish brown, or have an obvious grey rim. Their hair is ash brown, steely grey, ash blond or salt'n'pepper coloured, with no hint of gold or auburn.

- If you're an ice maiden, look at your favourite colour piles. Do they match the suggestions opposite? Does this explain why they suit you? If yes, check out the guidelines on the opposite page.

- If not, wait until tomorrow to try out some other colour options.

PLAY WITH COLOUR

Famous ice maidens include Queen Elizabeth II.

Colours to suit an ice maiden

What colours suit you?

 These are your best colours for coats, formal suits, shoes, bags and belts. These are your wardrobe basics.

 Pure white is good if you are tanned, or soft white if you are pale. Silver and platinum jewellery positively sparkles.

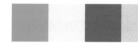

These are great colours to mix and match with. Use them for clothes, make-up and accessories.

How should you wear your favourite colours?

Always combine your favourite colours with other colours that have a cool undertone.

Colours that kill

Your worst colours are those with a warm, golden quality. If you can't avoid them, make sure you wear cooler shades next to your face and try to blend cool and warm shades in the same colour – for example, coral works with raspberry. If you wear gold jewellery, make sure it's shiny and sparkles.

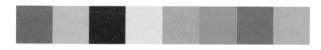

PLAY WITH COLOUR

How bold are you?

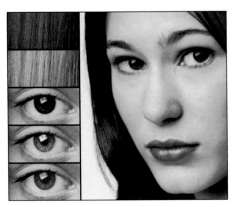

If you're still unsure, maybe undertone is not the most important thing for you. Today we'll look at the intensity of a colour to see if you can wear bright, vibrant colours.

Activity

Are you bold and bright

- Look again at your reflection in the mirror. Is there a great deal of contrast in your colouring? For example, have you got really dark hair and pale skin? If so, perhaps you are one of those people who can wear bright, clear colours and look fabulous.

- Now look at your eyes – do they dazzle and have a jewel-like quality? They might be blue, green, turquoise or bright hazel. If they do, here's a clue.

- Look at your favourite colour piles. Are they full of bright and bold colours that match the suggestions opposite? Does this explain why they suit you? If yes, check out the guidelines on the opposite page.

- If not, the next step will examine whether soft and subtle colours suit you.

PLAY WITH COLOUR

People with bold and bright colouring include Liv Tyler and Liz Hurley – or Snow White!

Bold and bright colours to suit you

What colours suit me?

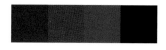

These are your best colours for coats, formal suits, shoes, bags and belts. These are your wardrobe basics.

You're a stunner in bright white. Sparkly gems and tropical coloured jewellery look fabulous against your skin.

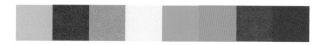

Choose jewel-like colours to mix and match. It doesn't matter whether they have a warm or cool undertone as long as they are really clear and vivid. Use them for clothes, make-up and accessories.

How should I wear my favourite colours?

Combine bright colours and aim for high contrast – for example, dark brown and bright turquoise. It won't look overpowering.

Colours that kill

Your worst colours are those in soft, mid tones that will make you look washed out. If you can't avoid them, wear bold bright shades next to your face.

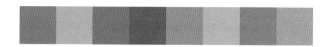

PLAY WITH COLOUR

Are you keeping up? Do you need some help? If you've not already subscribed, why not try the daily text messaging service for extra encouragement and support. Just text 'Fab 21' to 80881 now.

Each set of messages costs £1.50. Please see page xiii for full terms and conditions.

Are you soft and subtle?

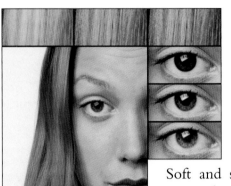

You must be getting a feel now for the qualities of colour that suit you. If wearing bright colours makes you want to reach for your sunglasses, perhaps you look best in soft, subtle colours that contain a dash of grey in the dye mix.

Soft and subtle-looking women who've got colours sussed often wear toning rather than contrasting shades, and look

Activity

Are you soft and subtle?

- How would you describe the overall colouring of your face, eyes and hair? If the overall effect is rich and dusky, you have soft, subtle colouring. Bright colours will look garish on you.

- Now look at your eyes – if they're soft grey, grey/blue, brown, olive green or hazel, this could be the colour tone for you. What about your hair – is it blonde, light brown, mousey or yellow-grey?

- Look at your favourite clothes piles. Are they full of dusky tones that match our suggestions? Does this explain why they suit you? If yes, check out the guidelines on the opposite page.

- If not, tomorrow you can see whether deep, dark colours suit you.

softly harmonious from head to foot. Of course, being soft and subtle has nothing to do with your personality – it's all about your skin, hair and eyes.

People with soft and subtle colouring include Cindy Crawford and Tara Palmer-Tomlinson.

Soft and subtle colours to suit you

What colours suit me?

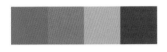 These are your best colours for coats, formal suits, shoes, bags and belts. These are your wardrobe basics.

Soft whites look better than bright shades. Mother-of-pearl and wooden jewellery looks good on you.

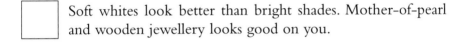

These are great colours to mix and match with. Use them for clothes, make-up and accessories.

How should I wear my favourite colours?

Harmonise soft colours and aim for toning shades – for example burnt copper and creamy yellow, or peacock blue and sage green.

Colours that kill

Your worst colours are those with a bright, bold quality. If you can't avoid them, try to wear softer, more subtle colours next to your face.

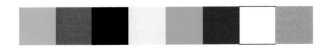

How deep can you go?

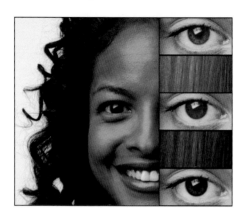

You'll know for sure if you look good in deep colours because your look will be predominantly dark. At least two out of three of your hair, skin and eyes will be deep. For example, you might have dark eyes and hair and medium-toned skin. Or you might have dark skin and hair, but blue eyes. Even if you have blue and green eyes, they will be deep pools. You will certainly tan easily and rarely burn.

Activity
Are you deep and intense?

- Hold the dark items from your colour piles – those with lots of black in the dye mix – up against your face.

- Notice what the deep colours do to your skin, eyes and hair. If you have deep colouring, these shades will really emphasise the intensity of your look. Lucky you – you'll look great in black. If not, they will drain you and give you shadows.

- If you are deep and intense (in looks at least), look at your favourite colour piles. Do they match the suggestions opposite? Does this explain why they suit you? If yes, check out the guidelines on the opposite page.

- If not, wait until the next step to see if you're fair of face.

PLAY WITH COLOUR

Famous people with deep and intense colouring are Halle Berry, Catherine Zeta-Jones and Penelope Cruz.

Deep and intense colours to suit you

What colours suit me?

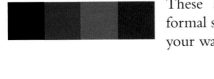

These are your best colours for coats, formal suits, shoes, bags and belts. These are your wardrobe basics.

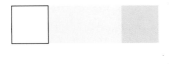

Your best white is a crisp, stark white. In addition, your dark skin looks great with crisp, icy pastels, providing you show off lots of dark skin, or wear them with other deep colours and vibrant make-up.

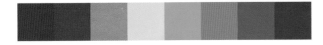

These are great colours to mix and match with. Use them for clothes, make-up and accessories.

How should I wear my favourite colours?

You can wear two deep colours together, or wear deep with light, bright colours. Don't be afraid to go for drama.

Colours that kill

Your worst colours are those which are both light and soft. They cry out to be mixed with deep, intense shades. If you can't avoid them, make sure you combine them with shades that do suit you.

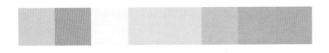

PLAY WITH COLOUR

Are you fair of face?

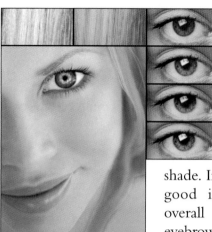

'Monday's child is fair of face.' Traditional rhyme

You may not have been born on a Monday, but if your colouring is fair, you will probably look best in colours that are a light to medium shade. If you dye your hair, you will look good in light shades, providing your overall look is pale. If you have dark eyebrows and deep eyes, this is not you!

Activity

Are you a fair maiden?

- Working in daylight and without make-up as before, find some articles of clothing that are light, pastel shades – with lots of white in the dye mix. Hold them up against your face.

- Notice whether the light reflects against your skin, showing up your eyes. If you have fair colouring, these light shades will really emphasise your look. If not, you'll look washed out.

- Now try a deep shade for contrast. Are you overpowered by bold, deep colours?

- If pale shades suit you, look at your favourite colour piles. Do they match the suggestions opposite? Does this explain why they suit you? If yes, check out the guidelines on the opposite page.

PLAY WITH COLOUR

Famous Monday's children include Paris Hilton and Gwyneth Paltrow.

Colours to suit a fair maiden

What colours suit me?

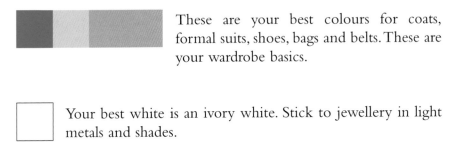

These are your best colours for coats, formal suits, shoes, bags and belts. These are your wardrobe basics.

Your best white is an ivory white. Stick to jewellery in light metals and shades.

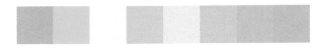

These are great colours to mix and match with. Use them for clothes, make-up and accessories.

How should I wear my favourite colours?

Always combine light colours with other light, pale colours.

Colours that kill

Your worst colours are those with a lot of black in the dye mix – you'll look like you're in mourning. If you have to wear a dark colour, wear it with a paler colour, especially next to your face.

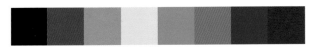

PLAY WITH COLOUR

Refine your colour palette

The last few activities have looked at the qualities of colour that work best for you. If you're still not sure, don't panic, help is at hand.

In this decade – the noughties – we're spoilt for choice. The biggest favour you can do yourself is to pare down and fine-tune your colour palette. Unless you have unlimited money and a personal shopper to help, it's too time-consuming and expensive to have loads of colours. By using fewer colours, you can build a wardrobe that looks great on you and is easy to mix and match, so it will be more cost-effective too.

TOP TIP

- Your pull-out colour card is a general reminder, not a set of commandments. When you dress or go shopping, take it out and see if the garment blends or clashes with the colours on your card. If it blends, it's good. If it clashes, chances are it won't suit you.

Activity

Try some new colours

- Using your findings from the last six days, identify which colour range works best for you. Is it warm or cool, bright or soft, deep or light? If you can't decide, eliminate those that look awful. From what's left, choose the colours you like the best and that go with the colours in your favourite clothes piles.

- Now tear out the colour card at the back of this book that corresponds to the colour range you've chosen. Pop it in your wallet or handbag and use it as a reminder when you are shopping.

- Start a list below of the colours you want in your wardrobe. Begin with the colours you like from your existing piles. Choose at least two neutral colours for shoes, bags, trousers and coats. Then add in your other favourite colours.

My favourite colours	List of what I have in these colours
e.g. teal blue, dark blue	T-shirt, flowery skirt, bikini, jeans, work skirt suit

- Hit the shops with a friend and try out at least two of the new colours on your list. Step into natural light if you can, to see whether they really suit you. Why not ask your friend to take a photo? Complete your list of up to six or seven colours in total.

PLAY WITH COLOUR

Banish black

Black: so versatile, sophisticated, slimming – what a myth! Black is OK for rock chicks, Isabella Rossellini and nuns – as well as for those lucky few with deep and intense colouring. For the rest of the female population, top-to-toe black is mostly draining and unimaginative. What a shame then, that black is back.

There is a saying that women who wear black lead colourful lives.

We beg to differ. Unless the cut and fabric quality and weight are tip-top, it can so easily look cheap, drab and vampish. For many British women over 25, a column of black can only be carried off with immaculate grooming and make-up, and exquisite accessories.

If you're a black addict, this activity is going to be a real challenge!

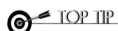

TOP TIP

If you have to wear black, make it more flattering by:

- Wearing it with colourful or bold accessories.
- Wearing it on your bottom half.
- Combining it with lighter, brighter colours.
- Avoiding it next to your face.
- Wearing a lower neckline.

PLAY WITH COLOUR

Activity

Step out of black

- Choose a colour other than black from your list of colours for wardrobe basics. Find one that lifts your spirits and flatters your colouring.

- Use the colour combination suggestions to put together some new outfits in your wardrobe.

- Step out with some friends and see what reaction you get. If they don't comment, say 'Do you notice anything different about me today?'

- Write down the positive comments you receive.

- When you get back home, stick them on the inside of your wardrobe so you are reminded next time you reach for that shroud.

PLAY WITH COLOUR

Colour camouflage

No - today isn't about wearing army fatigues! It's about how and where you use colour to flatter your shape. Anyone who's ever stepped out in a red dress knows that colour catches the eye and can make you look terrific - or like an overstuffed tomato.

Knowing how to create the illusion of a slim, sleek silhouette is the starting point to stylish dressing, and today you're going to learn how. Basically, there are two ways to do it:

1. Wear dark, matt colours to cover your worst parts and wear brighter, contrasting colours to draw attention towards your best bits. For example, use a dark top to cover a large bust and lighter trousers to show off shapely legs and slim hips. The only problem with this is that there's a horizontal break in colour that divides your body making it appear wider and shorter.

2. Wear one colour or similar shades from head to toe. Providing it's in a shade that flatters you and is cut stylishly, this one-colour style creates a long, unbroken line. It not only looks coordinated but also makes you appear slimmer. The eye glides over your trouble spots.

Today's activity is about creating slim looks from your wardrobe.

PLAY WITH COLOUR

TOP TIP

- The dark colour you choose doesn't have to be black. Look at the pallete of colours that suits you and choose one of the neutral colours as your dark colour – it could be deep plum, blue, brown or even khaki.
- You can use bright accessories to draw the eye towards your best features.

Activity

Look slimmer with colour

- Look at yourself in the mirror. Which bits do you want to divert attention away from? Is it your arms, bust, bottom, thighs or knees? Also work out whether you want to draw attention towards other bits. For example, you may have a big bottom half but really like your bust.

- Now you've done that, go to your wardrobe and choose clothes in dark, matt colours for your worst bits. Now team these with lighter, brighter colours for your good bits. See how many outfits you can make.

- Choose clothes of one colour or similar shades of the same colour. Now put together one-colour outfits and see what they look like.

- Ask a friend to tell you how you look. Perhaps even get her to take a photo – just for the record.

PLAY WITH COLOUR

Colours for effect

Now you know what range of colours suit you, the final piece of the puzzle is to consider the effect different colours can have on your mood and on the messages they send others about you.

In our western culture, some colours have definite connotations when worn by others. Consider these and see what you think.

Mysterious, chic, powerful, professional, funereal, austere, authoritative, severe, menacing.

Conservative, formal, perhaps a bit boring, depressing, efficient, reliable, neutral.

Confident, practical, stable, approachable, serious, boring.

Vibrant, powerful, scary, fiery, unpredictable, self-confident, dynamic, sexy, energetic, aggressive, angry, unstable.

Full of energy, fun, youthful, vivacious, stimulating, creative, restless.

Warm, glowing, sunny, optimistic.

Balanced, harmonious, hopeful, calming.

Knowledgeable, decisive, honest, dependable, sober, conservative, safe, stable.

Creative, visionary, inspirational, overpowering.

Pure, virginal, untainted, ethereal, stark.

Today you're going to observe the effect colours have on you and how you can use colour to lift your mood and change the way others perceive you.

Activity What does this colour say?

- It's coffee time. Get yourself into town with your notebook and sit where you can see people coming in and out or walking past.

- Look at the men and women walking past. For each person, note the colour of the clothes they are wearing – especially next to their face.

- What impression do they give? What personal qualities do they exude? If they work, what job do you think they do? What makes you think that?

- Do this for 10 people. Now look back over your notes. Can you see any trends about the effect colours have on you?

rson	o o r	mpr ssion o p op arin it
	ri t r	r ati i i rant s ar

- What can you learn from this about how and when to use colours in your own wardrobe?

PLAY WITH COLOUR

Your notes

CHAPTER 4

BEAUTIFUL YOU

Skin sins

What is beauty? If beauty comes from within, then when you feel good you look good. Making the most of yourself is key to your well-being as this will help you to build your self-esteem and project confidence. However, this doesn't mean spending a fortune – a few tips, some good habits and an understanding of what's right for you can make a huge difference to how you look and feel.

Your skin accounts for up to 12% of body weight, and of course it's vital in protecting your insides from the outside world.

The main aim of skin care is to maintain a healthy skin. As a healthy skin is a beautiful skin, this is really important in boosting your self-esteem. Whatever type of skin you have, the following is a recipe for super skin:

- Eat a balanced diet. Include vegetables, fruit, fibre and protein.
- Drink loads of water – about 2 litres a day. (Tea and coffee don't count!) This will speed up the body's ability to get rid of waste and toxins.
- Sleep. Skin repairs itself as we knock out the zzzs.
- Protect your skin. Moisturiser and sun screen are a must – even in winter.
- Keep your skin clean to avoid blocking pores.
- Exercise is great for the skin. It speeds cell production as well as minimising stress.
- Go easy on alcohol consumption and don't smoke.

TOP TIP

◆ Regular massage is good for the skin. It helps to nourish and revitalise, particularly ageing skin and muscles.

FACT: Sunlight causes skin cancer – only black skins have any built-in protection. In Australia children as young as 13 have died from skin cancer. Always protect your skin in sunshine.

Activity
Daily diary

● Keep a skin diary for a week.

1. How much water do you drink?

2. What products do you use on your skin and how often?

3. Are you eating a healthy, balanced diet?

4. Are you good at protecting your skin?

● Be honest with yourself. Identify where you could do better – and do something about it.

BEAUTIFUL YOU

Typical skin types

Until the age of about 30, your skin retains moisture and repairs itself quickly. After 30 it's less forgiving, so it's important to adopt a regular skin care routine. There are three golden rules of skin care.

1 **Cleanse** using appropriate products. Don't rely on soap and water as these will just dry out your skin.

2 **Tone** to remove any remaining grease and dirt.

3 **Moisturise** to retain water content and help your skin look smooth and youthful.

Although these rules apply to all sorts of skin, your type of skin will need a specific routine. Look below to see which type you are.

	Normal	Dry/sensitive	Oily	Combo
What's it like?	Clear. Not tight or greasy. Quite rare.	Feels tight after cleansing. Often red and blotchy.	Looks/feels greasy. Spots. Often dull.	'T' zone oily and cheeks dry.
How shall I care for it?	Creamy cleanser. Non-alcoholic freshener. Moisturiser.	Rich liquid/ cream cleanser. Very mild freshener. Rich moisturiser and night cream.	Washing lotion/milk cleanser. Astringent lotion. Very light moisturiser.	Treat as two skin types or 'combo' products.

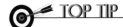

TOP TIP

- When cleansing, toning and moisturising, always ensure fingers move upwards and outwards. Your skin is a very delicate organ and can easily be stretched. For eye areas, move inwards towards the nose.
- Try your local college for a cheap but pampering facial. You'll feel great afterwards.

The secret to a flawless skin is always to choose products that suit you – your age, your skin type and colouring. All the activities in this chapter will help you to make those choices and will guide you to look fabulous rather than frightening.

Activity

Your skin type

- Using the table opposite, identify your own skin type. If you're unsure of your skin type or have particular skin problems, make an appointment to see a beautician or skin specialist for advice.

- Taking into consideration your age, skin type, skin condition and lifestyle, check the products you use and ensure they're the best ones for you. Chuck out any products over 12 months old.

- Your skin is precious. Looking after it now will reap rewards as you get older.

BEAUTIFUL YOU

Beauty basics

Whether you enjoy wearing it or not, your looks will be enhanced by a touch of make-up. Even if you don't want to apply a face-full, a few basics will give you a more confident, professional, youthful and polished look. It takes a little make-up to look natural, fresh and alert.

Start by checking your make-up bag. Essentials should include:

+ A foundation base or tinted moisturiser
+ Concealer
+ Mascara
+ Eye shadow compact
+ Lipstick that can double as blusher
+ Petroleum-free lip moisturiser that nourishes lips.

Your canvas

As an artist will prime her canvas, so you should use your foundation to give a smooth, subtle base. Aim for a fresh, light basecoat rather than a heavy artex finish. Generally, creams are suitable for drier or mature skins; liquids are lighter and suitable for all skin types; gels or tinted moisturisers are great for a very light coverage.

 TOP TIP

+ When choosing foundation, always try three different shades on your jawline – never on your hand. The correct colour will 'disappear' against your skin.
+ It's impossible to tell the right colour of foundation in artificial light. Take mini jam jars with you to the shop to bring samples home to try.
+ Do you tan easily? You may need a different colour base in the summer.

BEAUTIFUL YOU

Applying foundation is easy – as long as you blend. You can use a sponge or your fingers. Place a dot of foundation on your forehead, nose, chin and cheek and blend down and outwards. For an invisible finish, take care to blend along your jaw and hairline so you can't see the join. Work quickly to achieve an even look.

Handy hints

◆ Blend some foundation on the eyelids and lips – a great base for your colours.

◆ If your skin is crêpey under the eye or in the neck area, mix in some moisturiser to blend more easily in the creases.

◆ Concealer helps to camouflage the odd spot or redness. If you suffer with lots of redness, a green concealer will work wonders. Otherwise choose a shade to suit your skin tone.

The final step to creating a flawless base is a light dusting of powder. Translucent is best – it will absorb oil, help your foundation stay on and even out your skin tone. Dust downwards for a smooth finish.

Activity

Beautiful base

● Check your foundation is the right shade for your skin.

● Practise applying your foundation. Don't forget to cover up and dust down for a flawless complexion.

BEAUTIFUL YOU

Are you keeping up? Do you need some help? If you've not already subscribed, why not try the daily text messaging service for extra encouragement and support. Just text 'Fab 31' to 80881 now.

Each set of messages costs £1.50. Please see page xiii for full terms and conditions.

Blushing babe

Blushers add a healthy glow and help to define your face shape. Your blusher will add definition and balance your made-up look.

Colour

There is a massive range of blushers – both in type and shade. Choose one to complement your natural colouring. If you have a cool colouring, then bluish, pink, raspberry shades will look best. Alternatively, warm colours contain more yellow pigment and include coral pinks, rusts, peaches and orangey-reds.

If you have strong, bright colouring, then vivid blusher will look great. But if your personal colouring is softer and more muted, these vivid colours will make you look like a clown. Instead aim for subtle shades which will complement your natural skin tone.

If you have deep colouring, a strong, deeper colour will look fab, whereas if you're very fair try a light, pale pink or peach colour to emphasise your looks.

 TOP TIP

- ♦ If you apply your blusher before the eye shadow it will help you to avoid overdoing your eye colour.
- ♦ If you're out and are starting to look pale and wan, use a little lipstick as an instant blusher. Gently does it though!

BEAUTIFUL YOU

Cream or powder?

You can use either. A cream blusher tends to be easier to put on and looks fresher, although it can slide off more easily. If you've used a translucent face powder, put a cream blusher on before the face powder. If you're using a powder blusher, this can go on afterwards.

Location, location

So, where does blusher go? Apply it from the hairline, following the curve of the cheek bone and ending at the high point of the cheek bone. Alternatively you can just smile and aim for the plump bit. See which best suits your face shape.

Activity

Face up to it

- Check your blusher colour against your colouring. Does it work for you?

- If you're unsure, go into town and try different types of products and colours to see which suits you best.

BEAUTIFUL YOU

69

Eyes down

Your eyes 'are the window to your soul'. They are also the main focus of your make-up, so you can be really creative. There are a huge range of effects you can experiment with.

Two basic rules will help you:

◆ Light, bright colours draw attention and accentuate.
◆ Dark, softer colours help an area to recede.

This is exactly the same as using colours to emphasise or diminish certain areas of your body.

Activity

Eye eye

● On the eyes below, practise your eye shadow application using cotton buds as your paint brush. The steps below will help you.

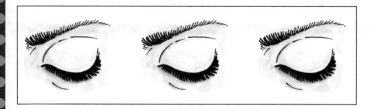

1. Apply a neutral colour or eye shadow base to the whole eye area. If you have warm colouring, aim for a warm beige; if you're a cool girl, go for cool, lilac tones. Base is great for keeping eye shadow on longer without creasing.

BEAUTIFUL YOU

70

2. Use eyeliner to create eye definition and fuller-looking lashes. Draw a soft line on the outer edges to make eyes seem wider. Ensure your pencil is soft and avoid stretching the delicate skin.

3. Choose your palette depending upon your colouring. 'Cools' should go for shades of grey, blue, pink or opal, whereas 'warms' suit browns, beiges, greens and golds.

4. The brighter or darker you are, the bolder you can go. A more muted or light colouring will look better in softer tones.

5. Where do the colours go? Your main lid colour should be applied first – usually a lighter colour, particularly in the centre of the lid area.

6. Darker, neutral tones should be applied along the lash line and crease of the eyes. Form a 'v' shape.

7. Apply highlighter above the wishbone towards the eyebrow area.

● Once you've got a look you like on paper, try it out for real.

TOP TIP

◆ Wear glasses? Ensure your eye make-up complements your frame colour and style. Heavier frames can take heavier make-up; finer frames require less.

◆ Black eyeliner is too harsh for most colourings. Try charcoal or brown instead.

BEAUTIFUL YOU

Lips and lashes

Lipstick is the easiest and quickest way to add colour to your face. Short steps to luscious lips are:

◆ Choose lipstick to suit your colouring – 'cools' should use pinks, reds and plums, 'warms' look best in peach, bronze and orangey reds.

◆ Use a lip liner to prevent 'bleeding', create definition and reshape lips. For a more natural look use a lip liner which is the same colour or slightly lighter than your lips.

◆ Using a lip brush loaded with lipstick, start at the centre and work outwards.

◆ Blot with a piece of folded tissue paper and add another layer.

◆ A dab of gloss in the middle of your lips gives a natural pout.

TOP TIP

◆ Get your eyebrows plucked professionally to make the most of your eyes.

◆ If you have very fair lashes and brows, try having them tinted for extra emphasis – especially if you're a water baby.

◆ Use a Vitamin E cream or petroleum-free cream to moisturise your lips, and remember sunscreen in the sun.

◆ Unless you're Catherine Zeta-Jones, stick to either bold eyes or ruby lips. Doing both is overkill.

BEAUTIFUL YOU

Use mascara to darken and thicken your lashes. Although it is available in different colours, brown and black are the most useful. Choose whichever complements your own colouring best. If you're very dark with dark eyes, black will look stunning. But if you're fair, a dollop of black mascara could make you look like a member of the Addams family.

If you have straight lashes, use magic heated eyelash curlers. Always ensure the lashes are covered from the root to the tip and use two to three coats rather than one thick coat. Flutter those lashes ...

Activity

Eye pamper

- Give your eyes a treat by using an eye mask to reduce puffiness and minimise any shadows. Used once a week, this can make a big difference to your very delicate eye area.

- If you don't already use one, then an eye cream is really beneficial used on a daily basis. Do not use normal moisturiser in this area as the skin around the eyes is much thinner than elsewhere.

- For a cheap fix, ice cubes will take away puffiness in minutes.

BEAUTIFUL YOU

Upping the ante

> 'Personal beauty is a better introduction than any letter.'
> Diogenes Laertius, 3rd century biographer of Ancient
> Greek philosophers

You will want to try different looks for different occasions. If you're a nature girl, then you'll probably be happiest with a more minimal look. However we all like to glam it up for a special evening out – and here's how.

Evening make-up needs to be stronger and probably more colourful. Remember, artificial light will dim your glory. In particular, go for eye liner and stronger eye colours, more depth to your blusher and stronger lip colours. Exciting colour combinations, gloss and even false eyelashes can add to your pazazz.

TOP TIP

♦ For a very special event such as a wedding, it is really worth booking a make-up lesson or even having it done professionally. If you decide to do this, do have a trial run beforehand.

BEAUTIFUL YOU

Activity

Face up to it

● Time for a treat!
Book yourself into a salon for a facial treatment.
If you're coming up to a special event, ensure
this is done about 3–4 days beforehand as the
skin looks its best a couple of days afterwards.
Even if there's no special event on the horizon,
go on – your skin deserves it.

● Be sure to ask for advice about ongoing skin
care, and if you can, book a facial for every 6–8
weeks. Not only is this great for your skin,
you'll feel so much more relaxed afterwards.

BEAUTIFUL YOU

Hands and feet treat

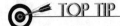

TOP TIP

♦ Never use metal files as they may cause nails to split.
♦ Use a daily foot scrub in the shower to prevent a build-up of hard skin.

Your hands and feet take such a pounding, they deserve to be pampered from time to time.

Whether you're image-happy or body-shy, beautifully manicured hands and feet will get you noticed and help you look polished. Take 20 minutes today to give yourself a home treatment. Although the skin on your hands is smoother, the process for hands is basically the same as for feet, except you can skip the filing off of dead skin.

Activity

Pedicure pamper

- **Prepare** Remove all jewellery and clean your nails using acetone-free polish remover. Soak your feet for 5 minutes in a bowl of warm water.

- **Smooth** Next, file away dead, hard skin with a buffer or file. Dry your feet and massage with a foot exfoliating cream to remove dead skin. Then rinse away dead skin.

- **Shape** Massage in some cuticle cream and leave for 5 minutes. Then push back each cuticle with a cuticle stick. Never cut cuticles as this can cause them to split and bleed. Cut each nail straight across with nail clippers. Round off each corner with a file and smooth any ridges with a nail buffer.

- **Moisturise** Treat yourself to a massage with aloe vera or peppermint cream, and don't forget to do your ankles.

- **Paint** Using dividers for toes, apply a base coat, followed by one or two coats of nail varnish, allowing time to dry between coats. If you're in a hurry and can't wait 20 minutes, dip your toes in a bowl of cool water to help your nails dry faster.

- Now repeat the process for your hands.

BEAUTIFUL YOU

Crowning glory

Or so it should be. Are you plagued by 'bad hair days'? On a bad hair day you can feel less capable, less good-looking, more embarrassed and less sociable. What an impact – and yet there are many ways to make the most of your hair.

Style sense

Choose a style which suits you and your lifestyle. There's no point in leaving the salon with luscious locks to find you can only achieve the look after 3 hours of spritzing, spraying and straightening every morning.

Horrid hair

There are several possible reasons for horrid hair.

Product promiscuity

You probably wash your hair over 15,000 times in your lifetime – imagine a garment washed this much! Choose the right products for your hair.

A shampoo which is too harsh for coloured hair will make it fade faster than a tan. Would you wash your hair with washing up liquid? Choose a quality hair product which suits your hair. When you shampoo, rinse off well – 2 minutes in warm water. Very hot water will make your hair more oily.

Be frugal with your styling and finishing products. Work them evenly through your hair, particularly in the root area.

TOP TIP

- Hair becomes very elastic when wet so always use a wide-toothed comb and comb starting at the ends of the hair, gradually working your way nearer the roots with each stroke. This will avoid breaks and damage.
- Talk to your stylist about the right products for you.

Nutritional nightmare

Eat a varied diet – often when your hair looks rough, you're not getting enough essential nutrients. Hair's the last on your body's list when it comes to the distribution of nutrients. If your hair looks horrid, maybe it's that crash diet? Consider some vitamin and mineral supplements.

Appliance overdose

- Always use heat treatment products to protect your hair from straighteners, tongs or your blow dryer.
- Use ceramic, not metal straighteners and avoid daily use.
- Blow dry from almost dry. Circulating air using your hands will be less damaging than 'spot' heating.

Activity

Heavenly hair

- Treat your hair by leaving in conditioner for 10 minutes. The hair cuticles will open to moisturise the inner hair shaft.

BEAUTIFUL YOU

Creative colour

Many women use hair colour to enhance texture, depth and shine. Women can feel different depending upon their hair colour – the boring brunette who goes blonde, or the mousey miss who goes red.

So what if you're feeling more grey than glam? Semi-permanent colour will help, or alternatively high- or lowlights will mask the offenders. When you find this disguise no longer works, a permanent colour will be more effective.

Complementary or killer colour?

The same rules apply as with cosmetics. If you have 'cool' colouring your most flattering hair shade will be cool, ash tones. Cool redhead? No problem – choose cool, red tones such as aubergine or plum. If you have 'warm' undertones, then opt for copper, strawberry blonde or warm chestnut brown. Always bear in mind that even if you were once a raven-headed beauty, as you get older you'll need to go slightly lighter as nature intended.

FACT: In the UK almost 80% of women use hair colour to improve confidence and looks.

Homemade or salon savvy?

Home-colour hair products are much better now than previously, although it's still very easy to end up with 'helmet hair' if you're not careful. There are certain advantages to home-coloured hair – mainly cost and convenience. Remember, though, looking like Alice Cooper for weeks isn't cool, nor is the cost of a salon repairing the damage.

Go for professional colouring, particularly if your needs are tricky. However, if you want to have a go at home, check out these suggestions.

◆ Start small – straight in at 'bombshell blonde' is a big step.
◆ Read the instructions – twice!
◆ Always do a skin/strand test.
◆ Put colour onto clean, dry hair.
◆ Wear gloves and protect your clothes.
◆ Apply Vaseline to your hairline to stop staining.
◆ Do you already have bleached hair? Don't do it – your hair will be so porous you can't predict the colour.
◆ Highlights are a salon job!

TOP TIP

◆ In between colour sessions, use colour gloss shampoo.

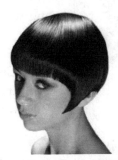

Activity
Colour crazy

● If your hair is coloured, take a look in the mirror at how well your skin tone and hair colour complement each other. If you look better with loads of make-up, then maybe your hair colour is a little strong.

● If you don't colour your hair, relying on nature may not be doing you any favours. Talk to your stylist about possibilities to enhance your hair colour and don't be afraid to experiment – just a little!

BEAUTIFUL YOU

Heavenly hair

Nothing is more important when thinking about your hair and looking great than the cut itself. The best person to advise you on this is your hair stylist; however, you may like to consider some ideas yourself before making a visit.

There are various styles for you to consider.

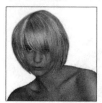

Bob Ideal for an oval or heart-shaped face. For a contemporary look, go for swing with textured hair.

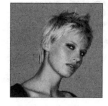

Crop Suits delicate features and petites. Again, texturing works well.

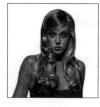

Long locks Can be either layered or one length. Layering gives body and movement.

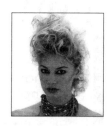

Curls Enhanced by layers which lighten and lift.

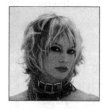

Shag Adaptable to different face shapes and great for wider faces. This choppy cut can be worn short or long.

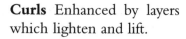

Further fixes

You may have followed all the advice and yet still have times when only a hat will do. Try these:

◆ Leave well alone – if you keep touching and fiddling with your hair it will lose its style.
◆ Use appliances – tongs, rollers or straighteners will help.
◆ Go easy on the lacquer – the Diana Dors look is no longer cool.
◆ Smell sweet – squirt a little perfume on your brush.
◆ Flat fringe? Dampen the roots and lift with a brush until it's dry.
◆ Put your parting on the opposite side from usual.
◆ Sunglasses worn on top of your head can be a really chic hair accessory.
◆ Scoop and pin up long hair with a few loose tendrils – sexy!
◆ Instead of going totally straight, use your straighteners to flick up the ends of your hair.
◆ If it really needs washing, pop your hair behind your ears and maybe slick it with some gel.
◆ Revive short hair by misting it with water and working in a little product from roots to tips.

Activity Memory lane

● Dig out old photos of yourself with different haircuts. After a good giggle, look and see which overall styles suit you best. Note how you've updated your look over the years and why certain styles look great.

● If you discover you haven't updated your look – it's time to do so. A new hairstyle will make you feel like a new woman. Talk to your stylist for professional advice – or find a new stylist!

BEAUTIFUL YOU

Smelling of roses

Personal hygiene isn't something we usually like to think about, let alone discuss. In fact, it's something only other people suffer from, isn't it? Unfortunately this isn't true. The problem is that we get used to our own smell so we're often unaware if we have an unattractive odour.

Whilst good personal hygiene doesn't make headlines, poor personal hygiene can be a massive turnoff and nowadays there is really no excuse for bad smells.

Help is at hand

The good news is that in most cases, a good diet, healthy lifestyle, regular washing and timely use of cosmetic products can eliminate or reduce most unpleasant odours.

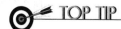 **TOP TIP**

- Always carry a travel-size bottle of mouthwash in your bag along with you. Most leading chemists now stock mouthwash that not only tastes good but also kills off the bacteria in your mouth that causes bad breath.
- Always carry some moist wipes in a resealable bag – useful for those occasions when you can't have a shower.
- Cure underarms and smelly feet with a quick spray of deodorant. Again, it's always handing to have some in your bag.
- If you're prone to smelly feet, wear shoes made of natural materials, such as leather.
- Treat your shoes to a thorough clean inside and out with a shoe mouse. Shops such as Lakeland Plastics sell them and in 10 minutes your shoes will be odour free. Finish off with some shoe deodoriser.

BEAUTIFUL YOU

Activity

Do the freshness test

You may want to do this activity in the privacy of your own bathroom.

1. Breath. Find a small plastic bag, such as a sandwich bag and blow into it with your mouth until it's full. Now close the bag. Wait a few seconds and open the bag, breathing in the air through your nose. How does it smell?

2. Underarms. We all perspire and modern deodorants help to keep sweat and odours under control, but sometimes we get used to our own smell. Take a whiff under your arms. If it smells bad to you, chances are it will smell dreadful to others. Remember, too, that clothes retain smells, so change and wash your clothes daily.

3. Feet. You know they smell if you daren't take your shoes off in public. Closed shoes and those made from artificial materials can be particularly bad as they don't allow air to circulate to your feet.

Your notes

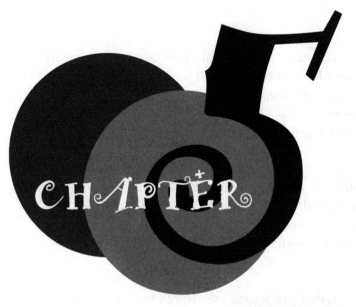

CHAPTER 5

SHAPE UP

Shape basics

It's true, colours of clothes and make-up can knock years off you and boost your mood, but the wrong shapes for your body can ruin your looks and self-confidence. Now you've got the right colours, it's time to pick shapes of clothes that accentuate the positive and camouflage the negative.

Do you remember, early in this book, you listed what you like and dislike about your body? Over the next few days, you're going to look at every aspect of your shape from top to toe. You will learn how to make the most of your assets and draw attention away from the rest. In particular, you're going to learn about:

◆ Your overall body shape, proportions and scale
◆ The shapes of clothes, from skirts to swimwear, that suit you best
◆ How to create a diversion so the worst bits don't get noticed
◆ How to achieve a perfect fit.

The good news is that you are the expert. No two bodies are alike and you know yours best.

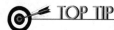 **TOP TIP**

◆ Have fun! Do today's activity with someone who will really give you an honest opinion about what suits you and what doesn't.
◆ Remember to look in your rear-view mirror!

SHAPE UP

Activity

What shape are you?

- Put on an outfit you feel great in because you know it makes the most of your shape. Perhaps it's one you've received compliments about.

- Take a photo of yourself and stick it in your notebook.

- Make a few notes in your notebook:

  1. Where is the eye drawn?

  2. How does this outfit flatter the good bits of your body?

  3. How does it disguise the bad bits of your body?

  4. What do you notice about the fit?

  5. What length is the top, skirt, trousers and/or jacket?

- Now do the same for an outfit that looks awful.

- What do you conclude about shapes that suit you and shapes to avoid? Can you start to write some 'what to wear' rules for yourself?

SHAPE UP

Are you keeping up? Do you need some help? If you've not already subscribed, why not try the daily text messaging service for extra encouragement and support. Just text 'Fab 41' to 80881 now.

Each set of messages costs £1.50. Please see page xiii for full terms and conditions.

Size matters

We live in a society that bombards us with images of waifs. Did you know that in today's sizing, Marilyn Monroe would have been a size 14? Models today weigh about 25 per cent less than the average woman. We believe that whatever your weight, this book is about making the most of who you are now.

> **FACT:** 38% of women in the UK are overweight. The average height for a woman in Britain is 5'4". Average weight is 10st 3lbs. Average waist measurement is 34", hips 40.5" and typical bust size is 38".
>
> Source: SizeUK survey, 2004

Hooray, then, for advertising campaigns like Dove's in 2004 that set out to celebrate real British women as people who are happy being different, normal sizes. Well done to role models like Dawn French for being proud of their size and curves.

So forget about squeezing into a dress two sizes too small and start by getting a hold of the facts about your shape and size.

 TOP TIP

- Don't assume a size 14 in one make is the same as a size 14 in another. Sizes are a guide and manufacturers all cut to different standards – so try before you buy.
- If the clothes fit you well but you hate the size on the label – cut it out! You never need be reminded again.

SHAPE UP

90

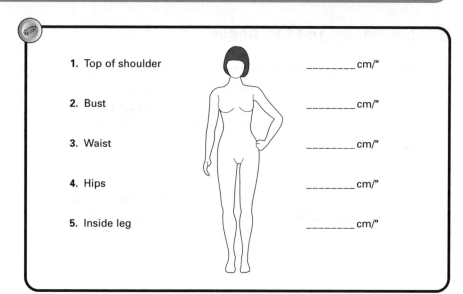

1. Top of shoulder _____ cm/"

2. Bust _____ cm/"

3. Waist _____ cm/"

4. Hips _____ cm/"

5. Inside leg _____ cm/"

Activity

What size are you?

● Use a tape measure to mark your vital statistics on the chart above.

● **Top of shoulder** Measure from the collarbone. Dress lengths are taken from the top of shoulder to the hem.

● **Bust** Measure around the fullest part.

● **Waist** Measure around your natural waistline.

● **Hips** Measure at the widest part.

● **Inside leg** Measure from the top of the inside leg at the crutch to the ankle bone.

● Use your measurements as a guide to clothes sizes when you go shopping (see the sizing guide in the Appendix at the back of this book).

SHAPE UP

Bottom-heavy and top-heavy

Let's start by getting a grip of your overall shape. Two shapes that many magazines refer to are busty and pear-shape. If you're shaped like Jordan, you are top-heavy and have a bust that is wider than your hips. If you're shaped like J-Lo, you have a shapely backside and a bottom half that is wider than your bust.

In each case, you need to use clothes to create an illusion of balance between your top and bottom halves. Check out the style rules for each type.

Bottom-heavy	
Do wear:	**Don't wear:**
• Skirts with flared and handkerchief hems to draw attention away from your bottom • A pair of slimming dark jeans with slanted back pockets • Jackets with wider lapels to balance your bottom half • Heels to lengthen your silhouette and slim your bottom.	• Boxy jackets and tight tops that will make your bottom look huge • Tapered trousers – unless you want to look like Humpty Dumpty • Bias-cut skirts – you need clothes that swing, not cling.

Top-heavy

Do wear:

- A well-fitted bra that lifts and separates – check the straps and make sure it gives you LIFT!
- V-necks and wrap tops with a camisole underneath to minimise cleavage
- Single-breasted jackets with narrow lapels
- Boot-cut trousers and flared skirts to stop you looking top-heavy
- Chandelier earrings to draw the eye away from your bust.

Don't wear:

- Anything double-breasted or boxy
- Polo necks – they'll make you look like you're carrying a tea tray
- Drainpipe trousers – you'll look like you're going to topple over.

Activity

Check out the magazines

- Get hold of a copy of a fashion magazine such as *Eve* or *InStyle* and look at the style advice for different body shapes. Even if it's not your shape, you can learn a lot by looking at others and seeing what they do right and wrong.

- See if you can add to the list of tips here.

SHAPE UP

Straight or curvy

Many would say that straight-shaped women are the lucky ones. If this is you, you may be a bit of a tomboy, slim and toned, with shapely arms, small bust, slim hips and an ironing-board stomach. What you lack in curves, you make up for in muscle tone!

Curvy women like Madonna and Catherine Zeta-Jones, on the other hand are rounded both top and bottom. If this is you, you have a defined waist and balanced bust and hips. You are the envy of all women!

In each case, have a look at what suits you.

Straight	
Do wear:	**Don't wear:**
• High-neck tops with cut-away sleeves to show your arms and hide your flat chest • Backless tops for instant sex appeal • Feminine, floaty fabrics, especially if cut on the bias • Pencil skirts that cling to the bottom • Diagonal and wrap tops to create the illusion of a waist and curves • Feminine jewellery and brooches – for a change.	• Very waist-clinching clothes that will be uncomfortable and accentuate your lack of curves • Baggy or straight-legged jeans that exaggerate the boy look • Deep scoop or corset tops that highlight your lack of chest.

SHAPE UP

Curvy	
Do wear:	**Don't wear:**
• Wrap tops and dresses to make the most of your chest and nip in the waist	• Circle skirts
	• Bags that sit on the hips
• Belted styles to accentuate your waist	• High-neck tops with lots of fabric around the chest, making you look top-heavy
• Low-waisted, wide-legged trousers to balance a shapely bottom	• Elasticated and gathered waists that bulge over the hips
• Flared-hem skirts to balance a full bust and elongate your legs.	• Tapered trousers – yuk!

Activity
TV watch

- Tune in to your favourite soap – perhaps one of the American ones with glamorous characters.

- Make a note of their different shapes and sizes.

- How would you describe their shape?

- What shape of clothes do they wear?

- Do they look good? If so, what are they doing right?

- Are they doing anything wrong in terms of clothes shapes that you can see?

- If you had to give one piece of advice about clothes shapes to your favourite TV character, what would it be?

- What did you learn that you can apply to yourself?

SHAPE UP

Tall or petite

If your dominant feature is your height or diminutive pose, today's advice is going to hit the mark. The great thing is, there's a style icon out there for every one.

If you're like Elle Macpherson, you're probably over 5' 10". Your height is an asset – all you need to do is create sexy curves.

Petite women like Natalie Portman are below 5' 4". Your motto is 'small is beautiful'. Make sure you choose clothes and patterns that suit your scale and draw attention upwards towards your face.

In each case, you can use clothes to make you appear less domineering or taller, respectively.

Tall	
Do wear:	**Don't wear:**
• Turn-up trousers • Soft fabrics and layered clothes – only the tall can carry these off well • Long cardigans – they won't swamp you • Horizontal stripes and big, bold patterns – because you can!	• High-waisted trousers or lots of vertical details, like pinstripes – you'll look like the Jolly Green Giant • Dainty bags – or you'll look like Harry Potter's Hagrid.

Petite	
Do wear:	**Don't wear:**
• Pinstripes and verticals that give the illusion of height	• Big, bold prints that will drown you
• Toning coloured bottoms, tights and shoes to add length to your legs	• Turn-ups on trousers, low-slung baggy trousers or flat shoes that will all make your legs look stunted
• Empire-line dresses that create length in the body	• Ankle-length skirts and bulky clothes that will swamp you.
• Small, delicate accessories and patterns that are in proportion with your petite shape	
• The highest heels you can walk in.	

Activity

Celebrity style clinic

• Look in a copy of *OK* or *Hello* magazine for your favourite style icons.

• Can you see people whom you know to be particularly tall or petite?

• How comfortable do they look with their stature?

• How do they dress to give that impression? Do they follow any of the style tips given here?

• See if you can add to the list of tips on this page.

• If one of them was your friend, what advice would you give her on clothes to flatter her shape?

SHAPE UP

97

Big and beautiful

If you fall into this group, you're probably a size 16 or over. The key to success for you is to make the most of the shape you are now. Female bodies are naturally smooth and their curves softened by fat. That's one of the facts of life that too many people try to deny. Here are a few style rules for larger ladies to follow.

Big and beautiful	
Do wear:	**Don't wear:**
• Make-up and ensure you are well groomed, to draw attention towards your face	• Tight cuffs or chokers, as they'll look like bondage gear and make you look bigger
• Well-tailored clothes in quality fabrics. They give a controlled yet feminine silhouette	• Polo necks, high round necks and double-breasted style tops
• V and scooped shaped necklines	• Leggings or pixie boots – either separately or together!
• Supportive, well-fitting underwear to help with posture and provide a smooth line underneath clothes	• Chunky knitwear, especially with horizontal stripes.
• Lower waisted trousers and skirts – preferably with side fastening and minimal waistband to avoid cutting across the stomach	
• Low-slung belts in toning fabrics.	

SHAPE UP

Activity

Online investigation

● Get online and type in 'image advice large women'. See what it comes up with.

● Read through some of the advice and make a list of your top 10 tips. Even if you're not large yourself, knowing what works for others can be helpful.

● Do you have a large friend? If so, what does she do well to make the most of her shape? Next time you see her, make sure you pay her a compliment.

SHAPE UP

Solid foundations

You don't have to be wearing an expensive and potentially jaw–dropping outfit to ruin it with the wrong underwear. You can kill a simple T-shirt with your saggy grey bra in just the same way. Here are some tips to help you find the right undies.

> **FACT**: 48% of women admit the main reason they don't wear most of their lingerie is because it's uncomfortable.

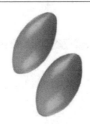

Chicken fillets
For girls with fried eggs, these are guaranteed to boost confidence. Try maxcleavage.com or figleaves.com

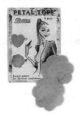

Nipple shields
If you're going bra-less but want to avoid the embarrassment of erect nipples, try Braza petal tops.

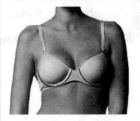

T-shirt bra
Every woman needs a smooth cup T-shirt bra in a nude skin tone. Never wear a white bra under a white top. Try Sloggi or Triumph.

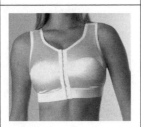

Sports bra
For breasts that need steel girder support, look for a sports bra with reinforced mesh technology. Try Enell.

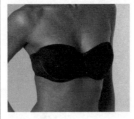

Strapless
Avoid the turnoff of greying bra straps under a pretty cami by wearing a strapless bra. Hanro do some good ones.

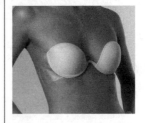

Backless
The ultimate base for backless dresses if you don't want to go bra-less. Try Rigby & Peller.

SHAPE UP

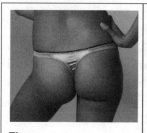

Thong
No more VPL with a thong. Hanro does a laser cut version – no seams or edges. Sloggi pride themselves on super-streamlining.

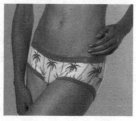

Boy pants and hipsters
Can't bear thongs and want to avoid VPL? These are the answer. Bodas have some fabulous ones. Especially good for shapely bottoms.

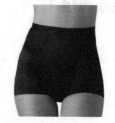

Magic knickers
These lycra and tactel pants will hold it all in to create a perfect lower body silhouette.

Activity

Get the perfect fit

Every bra manufacturer uses slightly different standard measurements, so here's how to check to see if your bra fits.

- The band around the body provides most of the support. Stand sideways to the mirror. If the strap rides up it's too tight. If it gives you back ripples, it's too small. If your breasts fall below your elbows, you need better support.

- The bra should sit flat against the chest between the breasts.

- Adjust the shoulder straps. They should sit snugly without digging in. If they fall off, tighten them.

- Check your cup size. Bend over to touch your toes (even if you can't reach!). Your breasts should stay in the cup and shouldn't spill over. If they do, you need a bigger cup size.

- Check the underwiring. It should sit under your breast without jutting out or digging in.

- Check the fabric. If it ripples across the cup, it's too big. Puckering at the nipple means it's too small.

- When you've found a style that fits, do the T shirt test. Pop a smooth T shirt on top. A good bra will sit smoothly and your bust will sit correctly and face to attention!

SHAPE UP

Tops and Ts

Fabric and print can completely change the personality of a basic garment. When it's worked with sequins, an unassuming camisole turns into a stunning party piece. Wear it with a formal outfit or use it to dress up jeans. Whatever your taste, start here with some basic shape essentials.

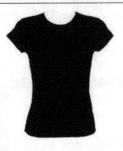

Basic T-shirt
Suits small to medium busts. Cap sleeves draw the eye upwards to well-toned arms. Balances full hips.

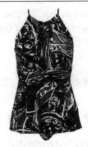

Halter neck
Adds width to chest and draws attention to square shoulders. Raglan sleeves do the same, but avoid if you have sloping shoulders.

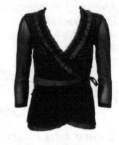

Wrap-over top
Flattering to a great cleavage and creates a waistline for boyish figures. Wear with a T, cami or halter neck.

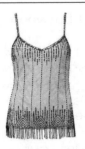

Camisole
Great under a wrap top or blouse. Adds interest and warmth.

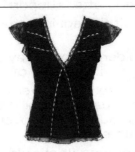

V-neck top
Suits fuller busts. V-necks divide and flatter big busts.

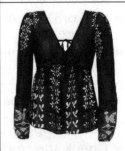

Fitted empire-line top
Disguises a round belly under the folds.
A straight top edge or slashed neckline balances pear-shapes.

SHAPE UP

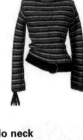

Polo neck
Suits pancake flat chests.

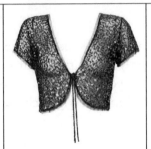

Shrug
Suits long bodies to create a layered look. Dress up or down. Try ebay for vintage wear.

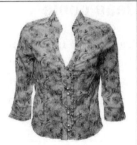

Fitted blouse
Creates a waist. Three-quarter length sleeves are especially flattering for wobbly arms. Try men's shirt makes like Ted Baker or Thomas Pink.

Activity
Eurovision top contest

- Invite your girlfriends round for coffee and ask them to bring a selection of tops and T shirts for day and evening wear. Get them all to wear jeans if you can, so the focus is on tops.

- Take it in turns to try on different styles of tops and dress them up and down. Make sure your neighbours can't see you stripping off as they walk past!

- Try different combinations and layered options and notice the effect. For example, put a polo under a sleeveless top, or a cami under an open blouse.

- Give yourselves marks out of 10 for each look: 5 for originality and 5 if it suits you. You could hold up your scores on cards. The person who gets the most points can have an extra biscuit!

SHAPE UP

Jean genie

Jeans – the most popular item of clothing ever invented. Sadly, it's not the most flattering unless you get the right style and fit. A great pair says more about you than your choice of partner, car or jewellery, so here are some tips for making the right choice.

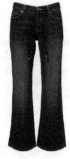

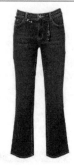

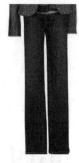

Bootleg/flared
Flatters most shapes, especially pear. Go for some fabric stretch. Looks worst on petite figures. Try French Connection.

Straight/slim
Good for boyish, petite ladies and supermodels. Otherwise steer clear. Try 7 for all Mankind.

Classic/relaxed
Great for pear-shapes and if you have chunky thighs and knees. A no-no for petite figures. Go for plain, dark denim. Try Diesel.

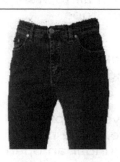

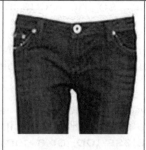

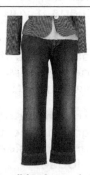

High-rise/tilted waist
Great for lengthening legs and for obscuring a long back. Can make hips and tummies bulge. Try Ralph Lauren.

Low-rise
Best for long bodies and lean legs, but **never** show your midriff unless you have an ironing-board belly. And if you have to show your knickers, make them pretty. Try Gap.

Sandblasting and embroidery
Great for tall, slim builds. Disastrous for big tummies and chunky legs. Try Earl Jean.

SHAPE UP

TOP TIP

- Always prioritise fit over trendy labels.
- For maximum leg length, the hem should be $^1/_2$–$^3/_4$" off the ground with heels.
- Cropped jeans look great on long pins but make everyone else look short, fat and dumpy.
- Wear cropped trousers with boots or delicate shoes – never with trainers.

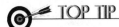

Jeantastic

- Get together with two or three girlfriends, preferably ones who share the same clothes size. Bring your jeans, shoes for different occasions, a handful of tops and a few bottles of wine.

- Try on each others' jeans and see what you notice about the cut, fabric stretch and weight.

- Notice what a difference each cut makes to your silhouette. Does it slim your thighs and hips? Keep on the ones with the best cut and fit for you.

- Find your favourite pair of jeans and match it with tops, shoes and accessories for a number of different looks.

SHAPE UP

Skirting the issue

Most women can wear skirts, but few do. Why is that? Is it for fear of showing their dimpled knees? With few exceptions, there really is a skirt out there to suit everyone. The essential things to consider are: overall shape, waist construction, fabric quality and drape, and length. Here are some suggestions.

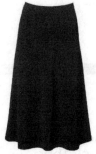 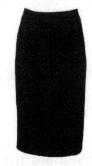 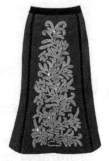

A-line and flared skirts	Pencil	Panelled skirt
Suit women with wide hips, full busts and chunky ankles. The wider hemline creates an illusion of balance. If you have a fuller tummy choose a skirt with no obvious waistband that sits at the top of the hips.	Very flattering if you have a shapely or big bottom. Make sure it's lined and that it's large enough for you to sit down in without it splitting.	Fantastic for creating the illusion of long, lean pins. Usually has a small or no waistband. Flatters rounded tummies. Good for straight-shaped women.

 TOP TIP

- ◆ To be sure you're seeing what others see of your legs, get a friend to take a photo.
- ◆ Avoid skirts that cut across the knee – you'll look like a rugby player in a scrum.

SHAPE UP

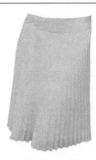

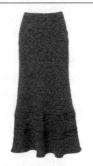

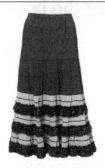

Pencil pleated from waist	**Bias cut**	**Tiered**
Great if you've got slim hips or an hourglass shape, especially if worn with a close-fitting top. The vertical pleats will lengthen your leg and create a very feminine look. Wear with feminine heels.	The fabric is cut on the diagonal. Great for boyish figures to create curves, but suicide for saddlebags – the fabric will cling in all the wrong places.	A good look for long legs. The horizontal tiers add bulk and will shorten legs, so beware if you're already on the short side.

Activity
Your ideal skirt length

- Wear a long skirt from your wardrobe or hold a large piece of fabric in front of you. Stand at least 5 m from a full-length mirror.

- Starting with the skirt reaching to the ground, slowly lift the hem so that more of your legs are exposed. Make a note of your ideal long-length skirt.

- Now raise it up. Your best mid-length skirt will finish either just above or below the knee at the narrowest point. Skirt hems should never cut across your calves or they will make them look chunky.

- How high can you go? Skirt length isn't about age, it's all about having fun. If you've got great legs and you want to show them off, go for it. Mini skirts with tights and boots can look fantastic well into your 40s!

SHAPE UP

Just the jacket

'Long hair minimizes the need for barbers; socks can be done without; one leather jacket solves the coat problem for many years; suspenders are superfluous.'
Albert Einstein, German born American Physicist

Einstein didn't put much store by personal appearance. But he was spot on in style terms – one good jacket can take you anywhere. Whether you're a one-jacket-fits-all girl, or collect jackets like other people collect stamps, there's a great range out there to choose from. Here are some of our jacket favourites:

- Bomber jackets look great if you've got no waist.
- Tailored jackets flatter curvy waists.
- Jackets ending at the top of the hip flatter most shapes.
- Mid-length jackets look great on slim thighs.
- Long jackets cover large bottoms.
- Jacket details and design can draw the eye upwards towards a beautiful décolleté, for example.

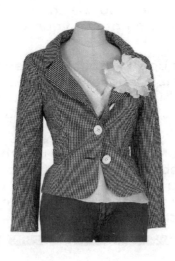

SHAPE UP

108

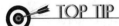

TOP TIP

- Long-waisted women should wear jackets that end mid-hip or lower. Cropped and short jackets that expose too much crotch are a real turn-off, especially when wearing trousers.

Activity

Jacket versatility

- Take your best jacket out of your wardrobe, even if it's part of a suit. Today is about making it work for you in a variety of different ways.

- Now choose a number of different style tops to try on with it – for example, a work top; a simple, thin pullover; a T-shirt top; and a fun one, perhaps with a draped or asymmetric neckline. If you wear dresses, see if you could combine your jacket with a dress.

- Work out a number of different looks using accessories such as shoes, jewellery and scarves. Try wearing the jacket both closed and open and see how it alters the style of the outfit.

- Make a note of the looks you like best and when you are next going to wear them.

SHAPE UP

Are you keeping up? Do you need some help? If you've not already subscribed, why not try the daily text messaging service for extra encouragement and support. Just text 'Fab 51' to 80881 now.

Each set of messages costs £1.50. Please see page xiii for full terms and conditions.

Coat cover-up

Whoever said a good coat will cover a multitude of sins was making a great mistake. The wrong coat for your shape can make you look more lumpy than lithe.

Here are some of our favourite styles. There's a coat here for everyone.

Activity Coat health check

Dig your coats out of your wardrobe and do the coat health check.

1. Do you have coats that fit for summer and winter?
2. Does the coat suit your shape and proportions?
3. Do the collar and lapels lie flat?
4. Are the sleeves the right length? They should cover just below the wrist bones.
5. Does the coat sag over your bottom or is the rear shiny from wear? Dry cleaning may help, but it may be time for a new coat.
6. Do the shoulders hang evenly? Can you stretch your arms in front of you without pulling too tight?
7. Are all the buttons and zips in good repair?
8. Is the lining intact?
9. Is the coat the right length for you? (See the skirt advice on Day 49.)

If you can't answer yes to all of these, get yourself sorted!

SHAPE UP

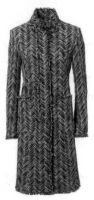

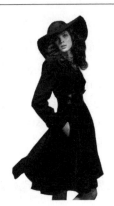

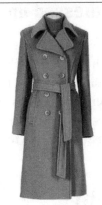

Slimline coat
Edge to edge fastening, hidden pockets and vertical stitching make this a great coat for petite women. Ideally this should end at the bottom to show off as much leg as possible. Discreet zip fastenings provide a slim alternative to buttons.

Tailored coat
Flattering if you have a shapely or big bottom. Make sure it's lined and that there's plenty of fabric to cover your bottom. These coats usually cost more as they take more fabric, but are a fabulous investment.

Trench
A favourite for slim, curvy figures who want to emphasise their waist. Wear it double-breasted to add width if you're tall and slim, or single-breasted if you've got a big bust. As an alternative, try a knitted, belted coat.

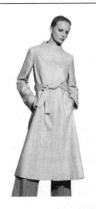

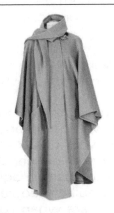

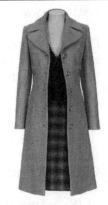

A-line/princess coat
Great for short legs. It hides where your legs begin, giving the illusion of luscious long pins. A wide funnel neck collar is great for flattering small bust lines.

Wrap or swing coat
A lovely wrap coat can be flattering for larger ladies and can hide a round tummy. Beware – these often have raglan sleeves, which only suit square shoulders.

Semi-fitted coat
The open neckline is great for short necks. This is a super shape if you have a round tummy. Watch out for bulky pockets at the hips that add width.

SHAPE UP

111

All dressed up

There's a time in every woman's life when she needs to wear a full-length dress. Whether it's for a wedding, a ball or a black tie event, choosing a gown to suit your shape is really simple once you've mastered a few basics. There are four basic shapes you will come across. Once you've worked out what suits you, you can choose from endless variations to suit you, the occasion and your personality.

Activity

Muriel's wedding

- Remember the film about the young girl who was obsessed with wedding gowns? Well, now it's your turn to play Muriel. Get along to the high street – perhaps to somewhere like Monsoon.

- See if you can pick out the four different styles on the rails. How have they been adapted? Choose one of each and try them on. See what they do to flatter your shape and proportions.

- Does one style suit you better than the others? If so, pull out some variations on that style and try them on until you understand what really suits you.

- Even if you're not going to buy, take along some heels and practise walking up and down in the dressing room with your head held high. Capture that feeling of inner confidence. Do you feel like Cinderella going to the ball? Imagine you are walking into a room full of people and they all gasp at how beautiful you are when you walk in.

- When you leave the shop, try to take those feelings and thoughts with you. You can use them next time you go out to a special do.

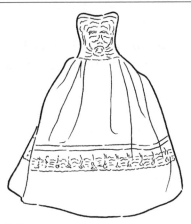

Ball gown

Traditional style with a fitted bodice and natural waistline that leads to a full skirt. Makes hourglass figures look disproportioned but looks great on pear-shapes with fuller hips. Imagine Grace Kelly in her regal attire.

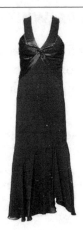

Empire line

High waistline right under the bust that falls to a slim or A-line skirt. Good if you have a short waist and longer legs as it hides where your top half ends and your bottom starts. Great too if you have a thicker waistline as it gives a long, slimming look. Petite women can look stunning in these dresses.

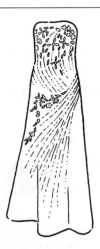

A-line/princess

Vertical seams flow from the shoulders down to a triangular A-line skirt. Classic and flattering for all figures. Suits hourglass and fuller figures, especially if you have full hips.

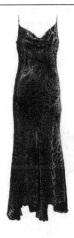

Column dress

The slim sheath silhouette closely follows the body line. Fabric is often cut on the bias so it shows every bump and curve. Only to be worn if you've got a figure like Halle Berry.

SHAPE UP

Flat foot or twinkle toes

The market for shoes has undergone a revolution in recent years. Even Clarks has gone trendy. Remember the recent advertising campaign to lure a younger adult market?

'Act your shoe size not your age.' Clarks shoes

Here's what we think every girl should own.

Office shoes	Dress-up day shoes	Evening heels
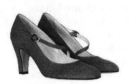	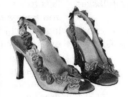	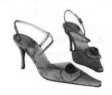
Straps around the foot rather the ankle are more slimming. Sturdy heels are better for thick ankles. Try Office.	Don't be afraid of shoe detail, especially if you're tall. Try Hobbs and Russell & Bromley.	Heels in the same fabric as shoes will give you super long pins. Remember, thin heels for slender ankles.
Trainers	**Going shopping shoes**	**Sensible work shoes**
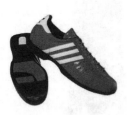	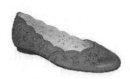	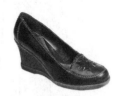
The go-faster stripe will lengthen and slim the foot. Try Adidas Shoshan, Puma Street and Gola Speed.	You could walk miles in these. Choose a neutral colour and they'll go with anything. Try Clarks.	Block heels are great for thicker ankles. You'll be well supported. Try M&S.

SHAPE UP

Everyday sandals	Holiday shoes
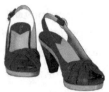	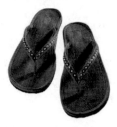
Open-toed block-heeled shoes slim the ankle and foot, giving the appearance of a slender leg. We love Dune.	Show loads of skin and create a long line. Suit most shapes.
Knee boots	**Sexy sandals**
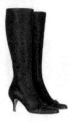	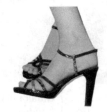
Pull-on boots give shape to fat ankles and calves. Super flattering for most legs. Avoid calf-length boots!	Strappy shoes add width and shorten the leg. Only for supermodels. We love Manolo Blahnik.

Activity

Shoe check

- A simple one today. Write in your notebook the different types of shoe you need, and write next to it what shoes you have.

- Do your shoes flatter your feet, ankles and calves?

- If they do, keep them and treat them to a clean and polish.

SHAPE UP

115

Bathing partners

When if comes to swimwear, we Brits have a lot to learn. Rumour has it there's a beach in Italy where style police can ask you to leave or cover up if you don't meet the beauty standards! So if you feel brave enough for a two-piece, avoid committing bikini sin and check out these favourites.

Triangle	Bandeau	Halterneck
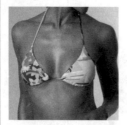	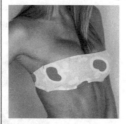	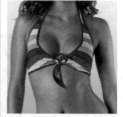
Small busts look pretty as a picture in these. Go for spaghetti straps.	Small busts look great in bandeau tops, especially with a bold pattern or horizontal stripes.	Great for small and medium busts to emphasise cleavage and flatter square shoulders.
Tankini	**Moulded and underwired**	**Gel-filled**
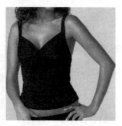	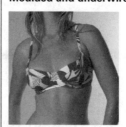	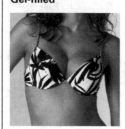
Great if you're long-waisted or want to cover a tummy.	For big bosoms that need a lift. Look for sized cups, adjustable straps and underwiring.	Great for creating curves up top. Super for boyish shapes.

In-between leg	Boy pants	High-cut leg / string
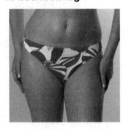	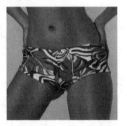	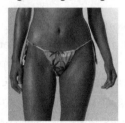
Most flattering – suits most people. Especially good for pear-shapes.	Only for the slim hipped. Can balance out a fuller bust. Shortens legs and creates curves.	Lengthens short legs but beware bikini lines and bumpy cellulite.

TOP TIP

◆ If you can't face shop assistants and hate struggling in a confined changing room, try shopping online. Check out figleaves.com.

◆ If your top and bottom are different sizes, choose from mix and match ranges from Debenhams, Monsoon, Oasis, landsend.co.uk, M&S and figleaves.com.

Activity
Two-piece tango

● Start by dragging your current costume from your wardrobe. Try it on.

● Compare the costume to the shapes described here. What shape is it?

● Does it work for you? If not, would you look better in some of the other shapes on this page?

● Get to your nearest swimwear retailer and try on different styles.

SHAPE UP

117

Costume savvy

If you're a serious swimmer or in need of tummy support, you're a one-piece girl. Shape, fabric, construction and pattern all play a part in turning you into a nubile bathing beauty.

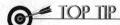 **TOP TIP**

- If you've had a mastectomy, the range of swimsuits is growing each year. Check out www.landsend.co.uk.

Moulded cups lift and smooth the bust

Wide-set straps balance full hips

Lightweight microfibre allows for quick dry

Ruching in cups adds volume and curves

Look for costumes with lining for support and to avoid those visible fuzz moments when wet!

A costume cut to the hip bone creates fabulous pins

Patterns and contrast	Visible seams	Wraps and sarongs
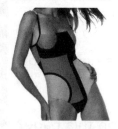	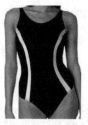	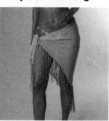
Patterns hide a multitude of sins. Bust-level stripes add width for pear-shapes. Darker, plain sections are slimming.	Shape the body and put curves in the right places. Great for fuller figures.	Great for big bottoms who want to cover up. Larger sarongs can be worn as a dress.

Sporty	Backless	Cutaway
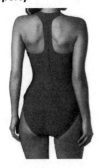	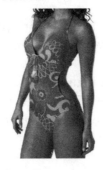	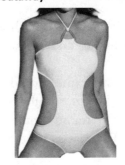
Gives freedom of movement for serious swimmers steaming up and down the fast lane.	Good if you want to distract attention from your bust and tummy and love a tanned back.	The latest trend. Only for super slim show-offs. Hopeless if you have bulges or want an even tan.

Activity
Siren watching

- Look in lifestyle magazine and find pictures of people in their swimming costumes.

- Look at all their different shapes and sizes. Which ones are like you? Which ones are completely different?

- Note what sort of swimming costumes they're wearing. Are they one- or two-piece? Can you tell anything about the quality or build?

- Pick out someone who looks good in her costume. What makes her look so great? Does she look confident? How much does her costume flatter her shape?

- What about your own costume? How does it measure up? Make a list of features to look for when costume shopping.

SHAPE UP

Spec-tacular

Whether you're choosing sunglasses or spectacles, there are four factors to take into account when choosing glasses:

◆ The frame should contrast your face shape.
◆ The size should be in scale with your face.
◆ The frame should repeat your best facial feature (e.g. eye colour).
◆ The glasses need to make a statement that suits your personality.

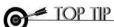

TOP TIP

◆ A long nose is best flattered by a low bridge.
◆ A short nose should wear a high bridge.
◆ Fat noses look best with a wider bridge.

Square face shapes	Round	Rectangular
 	 	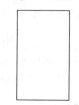 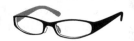
Think of: Sophia Loren and Emma Bunton (Baby Spice). Soften a square face with frames that are slightly curved. Choose frames that have more width than depth, and a high side position.	Think of: Stella McCartney and Dawn French. Wide ovals and pointy styles look great because they make the face look thinner.	Think of: Ulrika Johnson and Jade Jagger. If you have a long face or long nose, go for shapes with strong horizontal lines, thicker arms and possibly a lower bridge to shorten the nose.

SHAPE UP

Oval	Pear	Heart
		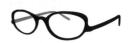

Think of: Sienna Miller and Penelope Cruz. These can wear most frame styles provided that the frame style and size is in proportion with the rest of the face.	Think of: Minnie Driver. Add width and emphasise the narrow upper third of the face. Try frames that are heavily accented with colour and detailing on the top half, or cat-eye shapes.	Think of: Jennifer Anniston and Sophie Dahl. To minimise the width at the top of the face, try frames that are wider at the bottom with lower arms, and rimless styles.

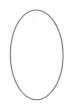

Shades to go

● Not everyone wears glasses, but we certainly all need a pair of sunglasses. The first thing you need to do is work out your face shape. The best way to do this is to tie back your hair and draw the outline of your face in the mirror with lipstick. Which shape does it resemble most closely?

● Look at the advice for your face shape. What kinds of glasses will suit you? Make a note in your notebook.

● Get down to a local department store and try on some sunglasses that work for your face shape. If you have eyesight problems, remember to wear contact lenses when you're trying on.

SHAPE UP

121

Blunder buster

You've reached the end of this section, which has looked at the shapes and cuts of clothes that will flatter your assets and help you camouflage your worst bits. Here's our list of the worst clothes ever designed to adorn the female body. There's no shape they look good on, so if you have any of these lurking at the back of your wardrobe, it's time to chuck them out!

1 Tapered trousers and leggings – they make the wearer look like a hot air balloon. If you have to wear leggings, save them for the gym!

2 Calf-length boots. Perhaps these were designed to skimp on leather, but they make most legs look stumpy.

3 Ponchos – best left to Red Indians.

4 Long, plain, shapeless cardis, especially if they've developed a saggy bottom through wear.

5 High-heeled white stilettos. Retailers have tried to convince us that this Essex girl favourite is now acceptable, but we're having none of it.

6 Visibly grey bras and underwear. If it's that old, it can't be giving much support.

7 A thong peaking out over the top of jeans. Unless they're jewel encrusted and you've got a derrière like Kylie, this is an invitation to hook you up by your undies!

8 Cropped jackets – only Stella McCartney looks good in them.

9 Boob tubes – unless worn like a camisole underneath a blouse or revealing top.

10 Wraparound sunglasses – unless you want to look like a wasp.

11 Mega platforms – even supermodels can't walk in them and they make slim legs look like golf clubs.

12 Unlined white trousers – VPL city.

13 Big patterned fleeces as featured on the shopping channels. They may be warm, but they're never stylish.

Activity

Chuck out challenge

- Read through the list. Can you think of any items you'd like to add to it?

- Pull out from your wardrobe any offending articles and give them straight to the charity, or better still, tear them up into dusters.

SHAPE UP

Your notes

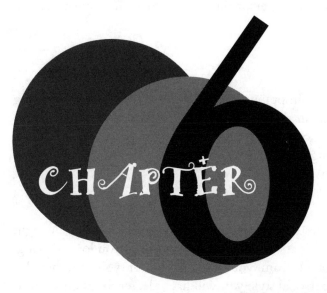

CHAPTER 6

PUTTING IT INTO PRACTICE

Who am I?

As well as knowing what suits your shape and colouring, there are three other things to think about when deciding what to wear: your personal style, your age (avoid the 'mutton dressed as lamb' look), and the occasion itself. If you weigh up these different elements, not only will you be able to tackle common dressing dilemmas, you'll also have the flexibility to let your personality shine through – whatever the occasion.

Personal style

Have you ever been shopping with a friend and bought something which looked great on the shop dummy but which you never wore once you got it home? Most women confess to at least one extravagant shopping blunder – so expensive, so stunning, yet it never sees the light of day.

This is because it doesn't reflect your personal style. There are no right or wrong styles. Style is about who you are and what you love wearing. This may be different from your best friend or your mother. By determining your personal style you will have clearer focus on what to buy and more confidence in how to express what is uniquely you.

Activity

Personality pics

- Take a look at these pictures and decide which set you'd be more likely to buy. Go with your gut instinct to get a glimmer of your personal style.

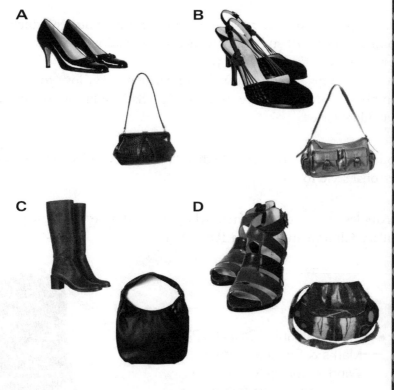

A
B
C
D

- If you preferred A, think 'Simply stylish'; B – 'Drama queen'; C – 'Au naturel'; and D – 'Creative chick'.

- As you work through this chapter, see if this is the case.

PUTTING IT INTO PRACTICE

Simply stylish

Yesterday's activity looked at your preference for shoes and bags. Although this was a bit of fun, often it is possible to see someone's personal style through the shoes they prefer and tend to wear. For example, you may have gone for **D** – comfortable shoes which are functional and fun – or **B** – the high fashion look. It's about what works for you.

The activities over the next four days will help you see which your dominant personal style is, or which combination of styles suits you best. Knowing this will help you to shop smarter. You will home in on those shops where you will find garments you love to wear. You can boost your confidence in knowing what's right for you and your individual taste.

Today you will discover whether 'Simply stylish' is an important personal style for you.

Examples of famous women who may fall into this category are Hillary Clinton and Isabella Rossellini.

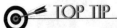

TOP TIP

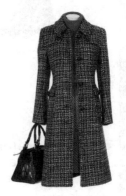

- ◆ Hobbs, Country Casuals, Planet, Marks & Spencer Autograph, Windsmoor, Jaeger, Cyrillus, Chanel and Louis Vuitton are some of the shops and designers where you can pick up this look.

PUTTING IT INTO PRACTICE

Activity

Are you 'Simply stylish'?

Tick which of the following applies to you.

1. You tend to be quietly confident rather than bold and brassy. ☐

2. You choose matching clothes and love to shop where there's a great choice in co-ordinated, quality clothes. ☐

3. You always look great. Your attention to detail and perfect grooming is the envy of your more slapdash friends. (You may not know this!) ☐

4. The suited look is very 'you'. ☐

5. You're organised with a flair for tidiness in the home too. ☐

6. You hate 'Dress down Friday' – a whole new wardrobe is required. What do you wear? ☐

7. You're uncomfortable with very casual dressing. ☐

8. You hate mismatched, badly co-ordinated accessories. ☐

9. You dislike a very loud, garish look. ☐

If you've ticked five or more, 'Simply stylish' is a key part of your personal style.

PUTTING IT INTO PRACTICE

Drama queen

Perhaps the last activity didn't particularly ring true with you. Today, you'll be able to see if you're more of a 'Drama queen' than 'Simply stylish'. Drama queens love to make a statement.

There are many well known personalities who go for this look – think of Sharon Stone or Victoria Beckham for starters.

TOP TIP

♦ For this look try Dolce and Gabbana, Moschino, Prada or of course your favourite designer. Wallis, Karen Millen, Episode and TopShop will give you good high street fashion to mix and match with your designer pieces.

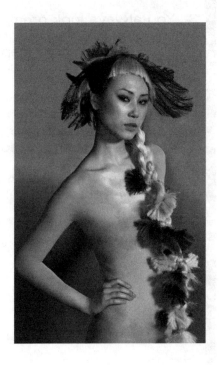

PUTTING IT INTO PRACTICE

Activity

Are you a Drama queen?

Tick which of the following applies to you.

1. You're pretty confident and enjoy 'standing out from the crowd'. ☐

2. You accessorise with hip accessories and bags. ☐

3. You know what all the latest trends are – in fact you're a bit of a 'mover and shaker'. ☐

4. You love wearing bold patterns or blocks of colour. ☐

5. You own some key designer pieces. ☐

6. You hate being a wallflower. ☐

7. You wouldn't dream of wearing 'last year's key look'. ☐

8. Subtle dressing isn't really your thing. ☐

9. You hate playing second fiddle. ☐

If you've ticked five or more, 'Drama queen' is a key part of your personal style.

As you work through the next few steps, see who else you may be. If 'Drama queen' just isn't you – take a look at other style clues.

PUTTING IT INTO PRACTICE

131

Are you keeping up? Do you need some help? If you've not already subscribed, why not try the daily text messaging service for extra encouragement and support. Just text 'Fab 61' to 80881 now.

Each set of messages costs £1.50. Please see page xiii for full terms and conditions.

Au naturel

Are you more relaxed than ritzy? Perhaps so far you haven't felt that 'Simply stylish' or 'Drama queen' fit with your style, so today will help you decide whether 'Au naturel' is more you.

Celebrities who are likely to be 'Au naturel' at heart include Emma Thompson and Sandra Bullock.

 TOP TIP

♦ If this is the way you enjoy dressing, try Olsen, Gap, Boden, Red/Green, Fatface, Kaliko or Cotton Club. Designers might include Nicole Farhi and Ralph Lauren.

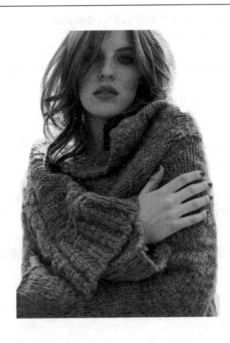

PUTTING IT INTO PRACTICE

Activity

Are you 'Au naturel'?

Tick which of the following applies to you.

1. Your clothes tend to go on your 'flubboard' (that's floor cupboard in case you haven't got one). ☐

2. Comfy and casual is where you feel most you. ☐

3. You might pop on a little make-up, but prefer the bare-faced look for a natural finish. ☐

4. Your favourite garment is your fleece. ☐

5. You're really into sports or the outdoors. ☐

6. You hate feeling uncomfortable in what you're wearing – you're not interested in tottering around on heels or feeling knicker-gripped by steel-like pants. ☐

7. You never quite get around to cleaning those shoes or going to the dry cleaners ... and as for hand washing ... ☐

8. You can't be fussed with lots of accessories – you can't see why anybody needs more than one handbag. ☐

9. You hate spending more than a few minutes getting ready each day – there's just so much to do. ☐

10. You hate very dressy events – the 'red carpet' is so not you. ☐

If you've ticked five or more, 'Au naturel' sums up your clothes style.

Perhaps you're a mix of this and another personal style – be truthful with yourself as no one style is better than another. It's about knowing who you are at heart – and maybe allowing the true you to surface.

PUTTING IT INTO PRACTICE

Creative chick

If you've not yet discovered which your personal style is, perhaps you're a 'Creative chick'. Today we will find out.

Alicia Keys is one celebrity with a 'Creative chick' personal style.

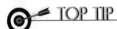

TOP TIP

◆ Try Matthew Williamson, Roberto Cavalli, Missoni or Alice Temperley to create this style. Or, on the high street, Per Una, East or Monsoon. Try pirateverte.com for accessories.

Of course, there are as many personal styles as there are women – if you don't recognise these four, try to describe your unique personal style.

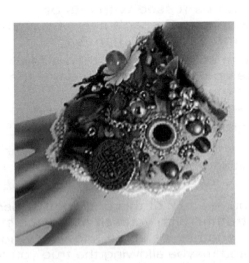

Activity

Are you 'Creative chick'?

Tick which of the following applies to you.

1. You really enjoy playing with clothes and make up. ☐

2. You're a 'shoe-aholic' – the higher the heel or the more unusual the better. ☐

3. You're comfortable being a woman and like to express your femininity or creativity. ☐

4. You like texture and are certainly not afraid of pattern. ☐

5. You're really into accessories – a girl cannot have too many handbags. ☐

6. You use your accessories to express your flair and style and add your personal touch to any outfit. ☐

7. You like pretty underwear. ☐

8. You hate 'boring' suits with no detailing or individuality. ☐

9. You just can't get excited by unadorned clothes. ☐

10. Flat shoes and trainers – no thanks! ☐

11. You're unlikely to go out and about with no make-up. ☐

If you've ticked five or more, 'Creative chick' is you.

It's likely you may be 'Creative chick' plus another – enjoy the best aspects of both! Use your creativity to express who you are through your style and personality.

PUTTING IT INTO PRACTICE

Different decades

Personal style may change with life events and age. Expressing your personal style is a must, whatever your age. But beware, what you carried off with aplomb at 20 won't look as chic at 40 – even if you are a 'Drama queen'. If you're not ready for botox and beige, what do you do when you're in the huge gap between Juicy Couture and elastic-waisted action slacks? This is an issue for many women as they approach their prime years.

The good news is that with age comes a healthier bank balance (supposedly) and also a greater knowledge and understanding of what really suits you. More good news is that you can express your style, whatever your age. Take care with some looks which really don't carry well across the ages – great in your twenties, not so cool now.

Take mini skirts, for example. If you've got the legs, these are great in your twenties and thirties. By your forties, you might prefer to wear them with boots and tights if your legs are still in great shape. But they're definitely out in your fifties. Although celebrities like Jerry Hall refuse to give up their minis, for most of us it's more flattering to wear longer skirts – just above or below the knee works fine.

PUTTING IT INTO PRACTICE

Activity

Mutton or lamb?

- Jot down in your notebook how you see your look. What gives you the edge? It may be your accessories or your 'classics', or is it how you keep abreast of fashion and update your look every season?

- Now note down what's great about being the age you are – both in the way you look and the way you feel. Be positive!

- Read on, the next few steps focus on great looks for every age.

PUTTING IT INTO PRACTICE

Triumphant twenties

In your twenties, your body's at its peak, but your confidence often isn't. It's a time for experimentation and personal growth. This is a time to find your fashion feet.

> 'If youth but knew; if age but could.'
> Henri Estienne, French bookseller and printer

A skinful?

OK so your skin's great, any pimples heal quickly and you soon recover from an all night rave. Don't take it for granted! Invest now ready for the future. You won't regret it.

Firstly, do cleanse and moisturise your skin – a light touch is the key here. Your skin will start to age from 25 years, so getting into good routines now is worth the effort. If you do suffer from spots, using the right products will really help.

Less is more when it comes to make-up. Keep base to a minimum and stick to light, fresh colours.

Navel gazing?

If you've got it, flaunt it. You can get away with so much now that you won't later – so enjoy. Got great legs? Be a minx in minis. Trim tummies on display or tiny bikinis? Why not? Enjoy the current trends by playing and experimenting. Above all have fun.

A word of caution – if your wardrobe only consists of minis, low-rise jeans, tiny tops and trainers you will need to 'dress the part' for interviews or going to work. Avoid too much flesh on display – perhaps add some shoes, trousers or skirt, a couple of great tops and you've got your gear. Hold onto your taste though. Use accessories and key pieces such as an up-to-the-minute jacket to make your statement.

TOP TIP

♦ Benetton, Miu Miu, Gap, Whistles, Oasis, Coast, Zara, TopShop and Marc Jacobs are all labels to try in your twenties.

Activity

Compliment a friend

● There's no better way to demonstrate your own self-confidence than to pay someone else a compliment. Take your best friend, for example. Think of at least three positive things to say to her and make sure you tell her next time you see her. For example, 'You've got great legs, you look fantastic when you wear short skirts.'

● Notice your friend's reaction. How does that make you feel?

PUTTING IT INTO PRACTICE

Tantalising thirties

The thirties are all about making decisions. From a style point of view, you may have made a few mistakes, but now you know what suits – don't you? You still have the looks and now you have the confidence to seize opportunities as they present themselves.

'It's never too late to be what you might have been.'
George Eliot, Victorian writer

Hello hydration

What you do to your skin now will make a huge difference in the future – cleanse, tone, moisturise ... and moisturise. Eye cream works wonders – say no to laughter lines. Drink up to eight glasses of water each day.

Your make-up basics will include a base, and even Cameron Diaz uses concealer for spots and shadows. Lipstick or gloss will be great.

Seriously savvy

This is the time to really start investing in your wardrobe. Know what suits you and create your own style. Invest in separates and buy one or two really great pieces – a sharp pair of trousers or fabulous jacket. Be fashion savvy not a fashion victim. You can develop style confidence and remain up to date by investing in some trendy accessories. Don't worry about every new trend that comes along.

Has your life changed or your body morphed? This doesn't mean that baggy sweatshirts become your uniform. Use foundation garments for any bumpy lumpy bits and seek advice if you're losing your style know-how. Now is the time to play to your strengths – legs, bust, waist, whatever. Pick the part you want to emphasise and flaunt it.

PUTTING IT INTO PRACTICE

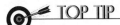

TOP TIP

◆ Miu Miu, Gap, Whistles, French Connection, Coast, Oasis, Zara, Reiss are all labels to try in your thirties.

Makeover magic

● If you're in your thirties, give yourself a makeover.

● Take photos of yourself in different outfits. What's great and what needs blitzing?

● Using the advice tips above, look through magazines or surf the internet and jot down three steps to a more triumphant or tantalising you.

● Do this even if you're not in your thirties, but work with a friend or relative who is. Give each other constructive, helpful feedback and support.

PUTTING IT INTO PRACTICE

Feisty forties

Not yet ready for beige boredom? This is a time to enjoy being grown up – no need to borrow your mother's pearls. Create your own fashion moments – be bold, glam and elegant.

Help is at hand

You'll now start to see changes to your skin texture. Maybe larger pores, deeper creases, your pillow marks stay with you until nearly lunch ... Keep hydrating – use cleansers, moisturisers, eye creams and drink lots of H_2O. Choose your products carefully.

Don't be afraid of colour – it's more important than ever. It's not all khaki brown from here. As your natural pigments start to fade, you may find that you need to soften your look. Muted textures and fur trims work wonders on tired complexions – like Vaseline on a lens.

Sizzling style

Invest in some 'hot' pieces. These will work with your more classic garments to keep you fashion-forward and trendy. Remember, you're like Liz Hurley – 40 not 80. Some killer heels and sexy underwear will do wonders for your self-esteem, and worn tastefully will get you all the right sorts of attention.

As Madonna approaches her late forties, take a leaf from her book and make the most of clever tailoring to flatter your shape. If your arms, tummy or cleavage show signs of age, go for shapes and styles that camouflage and draw attention towards your best bits.

Above all, don't descend into shapeless, appliquéd apathy. Rumour has it that women are at their sexiest past 40. You can still do sexy. Show a little cleavage; high heels and defined lips; a cropped cardigan or jacket with great jeans – get the idea?

PUTTING IT INTO PRACTICE

♦ Try Karen Millen, Aquascutum, East, Planet, Principles, Wallis, Hobbs, Fendi, Gucci and Prada for grown-up style.

Activity

Hello Mrs Robinson

● Remember smouldering Anne Bancroft aka Mrs Robinson in the film *The Graduate*? She exuded sex appeal because she was a confident older woman.

● What better way to feel good about yourself than to put on some fabulous underwear? Take a look in your underwear draw. Is it full of Bridget Jones big pants? Every woman needs at least one set of traffic-stopping lingerie. Even if you've got no one to show it to – wearing it will make you feel great.

● Perhaps it's time to go shopping with a girlfriend and treat yourself to a pair of outrageous undies. Try Agent Provocateur.

PUTTING IT INTO PRACTICE

Fantastic fifties and beyond

Older women just get better and better. Look at Lulu, Sharon Stone and Kim Basinger. They have more spending power, are sexier, more aware, healthier, fitter than previous generations of women have ever been at that age.

> **FACT**: A recent poll showed that 95% of women over 50 love dressing up for a night out.

Time for TLC

Your skin is now more sensitive, developing fine lines which will deepen. Less oestrogen means the skin becomes thinner and more fragile, losing its 'bounce back' ability. It's not all bad news as the right products will help you fight ageing. Invest in a gentle toner, rich cleanser, moisturiser, eye cream and night cream.

Make-up?

Choose the right shade of lighter foundation. Your colouring may soften – complement this with make-up colours and avoid metallic or glitter eye colours. Eyelash curlers, tinted lashes and brows (not too dark) will work. Apply powder sparingly – powdery creases aren't fetching. Plump up lips with medium depth colours, applied using a lip brush and pencil. Enjoy updating and creating your own look.

Essential elegance

Know yourself – create a look which is stylish rather than just fashionable. You may need more coverage in the tummy and upper arm department, but you can still dress with elegance and style. Ensure whatever you wear has a great cut and fits you well – no more tight-fitting Ts though. A slightly looser cut, wider trouser and details to draw the eye will do the trick. Flats are good, but heels look even better. Don't forget a new haircut and fabulous accessories too.

PUTTING IT INTO PRACTICE

TOP TIP

+ By the time you've reached your fifties, you probably have a strong sense of personal style. Don't be afraid to show it. And if you've discovered a great boutique, share your secret with a friend.

+ Dare yourself to visit 'young' shops like New Look or Miss Selfridge. You might be surprised at how a few, well chosen garments and accessories, worn stylishly with your wardrobe staples, can take years off your look.

Activity

Escape the rut – time to move on

● Now you're 50, it's likely that there have been significant changes to your lifestyle. But has your image kept up with the person you are now and the life you lead?

● Jot down in your notebook five words that sum up how you'd like to lead your life in your fifties. For example, outdoors, socialising, sexy ...

● Now flick through magazines and catalogues. Pick out some clothes or looks that are totally new and will meet your lifestyle needs. Next time you're out, try something new.

PUTTING IT INTO PRACTICE

Dress down dilemma

Are there certain occasions or life events that leave you with a wardrobe full of clothes and nothing to wear? The next few activities will guide you through these.

> **FACT**: Over two-thirds of employers now have a formal policy on staff clothing.
>
> Source: IRS Employment Review

These days, dressing for work isn't as simple (or boring – depending upon your personality) as a suit. 'Dress down' or 'smart casual' has come ... and also gone in some organisations. Dress codes are no longer as easy as once upon a time. The bottom line with 'dress down' days is that a certain dress code still exists.

Dressing down really does give you the chance to be creative. To dress down but still look like the boss try out these.

♦ Keep some structure and layer your clothes. A casual jacket or fine knit cardigan will help.
♦ Wear tailored shapes in more relaxed fabrics like leather or suede.
♦ Use colour to help you look more or less serious. Black, navy, grey, all mean serious business. Brown, camel, khaki are more approachable.
♦ Keep your accessories less formal. Your shoes, bag, briefcase should all tell the same story.
♦ Wear a jacket and trousers rather than a suit.

TOP TIP

To avoid dress down disaster:

♦ You should groom for success – dirty shoes or chipped nail varnish won't impress anyone.

♦ Keep flesh under wraps – no bum-clinging, cleavage-flaunting, belly-busting outfits.

♦ Save T-shirts with logos for the beach.

♦ Strappy sandals and bare legs should be saved for holidays.

♦ Torn denims are more 'rock chick' than 'office chic'.

♦ Floppy, flowery, ultra-girly clothes won't give you the edge.

♦ Dangly earrings, layered necklaces, charm bracelets and a beach bag may be over the top – accessorise appropriately.

Activity
Create casual chic

● Pull together a 'dress down' outfit which you could wear for work. If you wear uniform or do unpaid work, think about casual clothes which you could take on a weekend away or similar event.

● List the accessories/garments you need and add them to your shopping list. Remember to use what you already own too.

PUTTING IT INTO PRACTICE

147

Fab formal

There will be occasions when you need to dress more formally for work – or perhaps your firm has a serious dress code.

It is estimated that around 40% of senior managers expect their teams to dress formally. And what do you do for those interviews? How formal is formal?

You can create immediate formality through the colours you wear. If you partner a dark suit or jacket with a plain, light shirt or top, this high contrast look will be more formidable than a soft green, subtly blended ensemble.

A more tailored look with subtle, business-like accessories will all add to your ensemble (think smart shoes, Gucci watch, discreet jewellery neat bag, rather than high stiletto boots, chunky tribal beads or every trend of the season worn at once). It goes without saying that your grooming should also be impeccable.

Activity

Grooming audit

- Check your grooming is spot on – nails, hair, de-fuzz legs, pluck eyebrows, clean shoes, repair clothes, etc. Make a real effort to sharpen your image – today and on a regular basis.

PUTTING IT INTO PRACTICE

Interview ensemble

'You never get a second chance to make a good first impression.'
Popular saying

> **FACT**: People judge you based on what they see within seconds of that first meeting. From the moment you walk in, everything about your appearance needs to give off the right messages about your professionalism, reliability, quality, creativity, attention to detail and so on.

Don't let your image put a prospective employer off you. Never mind if you're currently a receptionist and you're going for the boss's job. Dress for the job you want, not the one you've got. Remember Melanie Griffith in the film *Working Girl?*

If in doubt, wear a suit.

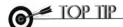
TOP TIP

- Do your homework so you **look** like you'll fit in.
- Attention to the little things really matters – clean shoes, tidy nails, great hair, polished make-up. Be neat, tidy and clean all round.
- Invest in a suit or look which makes you feel special.
- Carry any papers in a suitable briefcase or folder. Tuck a small handbag into your briefcase for an uncluttered look.
- Arrive early. You'll never look great if you rush in late!

PUTTING IT INTO PRACTICE

Yummy mummy

Pregnant pause

Bumpy doesn't have to mean frumpy. Don't let your style gurgle down the plughole faster than dirty dishwater just because you're pregnant.

Some women swear by raiding their partner's wardrobe – big sweatshirts or checked shirts create the look, perhaps worn with a pair of elasticated polyester slacks or even worse, leggings. Yuk!

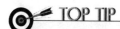

TOP TIP

♦ Check out great maternity lines, or versatile clothes you can still wear when pregnant: Formes, Isabella Oliver, Diane von Furstenberg, pushmaternity.com, serendipity-online.com, TopShop. And for jeans, look for 7 for all Mankind, Earl and Citizens of Humanity.

Even if parts of you 'bloom' like never before you can still look great, and you don't have to buy a whole new wardrobe to do it. A few key pieces will see you through. Here are some suggestions.

- ♦ Extra-long vest tops. If you're young and carefree, show off that bump à la Kate Winslet.
- ♦ Designer stretch jeans that feel great and look stylish.
- ♦ A wrap dress to show off your fabulous cleavage (go for it now, girl)!
- ♦ Slim ankles still? Flaunt them for all to see with beautiful shoes.
- ♦ Jewellery and accessories that make you look like a woman even if you feel like a bloated balloon.
- ♦ Look after yourself. Lots of sleep (don't forget afternoon naps) and take all over care of your skin.

Whether you buy from shops, online or a catalogue, remember that what doesn't normally suit you still won't when you have a bump. So if you normally have an ample rear, forget tiered skirts or jump suits. If you have a full bosom, it will become **much** fuller so forget large florals or horizontal striping.

Busy mum

The bump's gone, but where did you go? Life can be so full, so busy – having children is a full-on, unpaid occupation. Any spare money goes on the kids, you feel 10 years older than you actually are. If this is you it's time to chill out.

Activity

Chill time

Choose at least two of these suggestions and enjoy!

- Do a deal – swap services with another mum for a whole day and spend some time to yourself.

- Treat yourself to an image update – it doesn't need to cost much. Buy a few accessories.

- Cull your make-up. Buy two new exciting items.

- Chuck out any clothes which make you feel frumpy.

- Plan to have a lie-in – tea, toast and Sunday papers.

- Book a babysitter 1 hour early. Pamper yourself getting ready. Get ready to rock not ready to drop.

PUTTING IT INTO PRACTICE

Are you keeping up? Do you need some help? If you've not already subscribed, why not try the daily text messaging service for extra encouragement and support. Just text 'Fab 71' to 80881 now.

Each set of messages costs £1.50. Please see page xiii for full terms and conditions.

Socialite

You're invited to a posh do. Do you stress about your dress? It's important to get it right as dressing inappropriately can make you feel as uncomfortable as Lady Docker at a car boot sale. Be aware of dress codes and break the rules at your peril – unless you're a celebrity!

 TOP TIP

+ If you've got an event coming up and you're not sure what goes, then ask. It's better to do this and feel great, than worry about it and still get it horribly wrong.

Weddings

Often the invitation will tell you how formally to dress. For 'day to evening' you can do a tailored look such as a great trouser suit, or pretty florals. Anything too revealing in the arm area should be covered with a cardigan or jacket until the party gets going. Be as pretty as a picture if you wish. Hats are not necessary but good fun, although gloves are a bit over-the-top. All colours go, with the exception of black for daytime dos, and white (unless you're the one walking up the aisle).

The races

Generally, smart attire is the thing. In the Royal Enclosure at Ascot *'ladies are required to wear formal day dress and a hat that covers the crown of the head'*. Although elsewhere things might not be so strict, a hat is a must and too much flesh is out. Trouser suits are OK, but must be full length and of matching material.

> **FACT:** In 2002, Rod Stewart and Penny Lancaster were turned away from the Royal Enclosure. Rod's blue suit and white shoes and Penny's mini didn't cut the mustard.

Black tie

Long or short cocktail dresses are OK, even dressy trousers. However if it's 'white tie', long dresses are a must. Get waxing, plucking and faux tanning as flesh is called for at any posh 'do' – décolletage, an expanse of back or bare arms will look good. Heels are a must – no comfortable flatties whatever your personality.

School reunion

Forget playing it cool, you will want to look your best. Plan ahead to get the right outfit, and remember hair and beauty treatments too. Generally, these events are quite dressed up – so a Little Black Dress would be good or a dressy trouser suit. Avoid trying to dress younger than your age – these people do know your real age after all. Rely on quality, styles and colours which flatter you, and fantastic accessories of course.

Dinner at a friend's, colleague's or neighbour's

No particular etiquette here, other than to be comfortable but still look like you've made an effort for your hostess/host. Exactly what you wear will depend upon location, time of day, event, etc. Find out what you can and plan your outfit – then relax and enjoy.

Activity

Party planning

- Next time you're invited to a 'do,' plan in advance. Decide on your look and any rules of etiquette. Review what you already have and plan to buy accordingly. Remember dress agencies, friends or hire shops if you'd prefer not to invest for the long term.

PUTTING IT INTO PRACTICE

Your notes

....

....

....

....

....

....

....

....

....

....

....

....

....

....

....

....

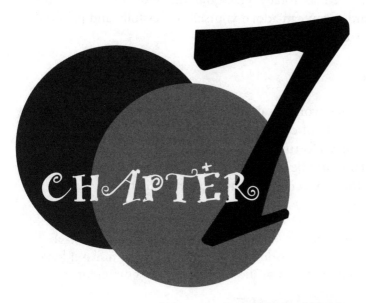

CHAPTER 7

**KEEPING
CURRENT**

Accent with accessories

You may love accessories and look for any opportunity to add to your vast collection. Alternatively you may possess only one handbag and one pair of earrings. Whoever you are, don't underestimate the power of accessorising. Accessories can create personal style and update your appearance as well as totally changing the look of your outfit. It needn't be hard – you can adorn yourself successfully and painlessly – whatever your budget.

Less is more

Many women are worried about overdoing accessories and usually they err on the side of caution rather than risk overdoing it. Are you working the 'hippy/fortune teller' look, or are you frightened that a bracelet too far could be your undoing? If you think you might wear too many or too few accessories, try today's activity as a guide.

'Belts, scarves, beads, bangles. Not all at the same time, but just one of these can add enough to an outfit to make it look 'thought out' rather than thrown on.' Anonymous

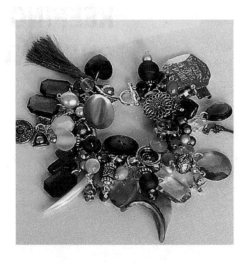

KEEPING CURRENT

Activity

How much is too much?

Look at this list and award yourself a star for any you're wearing right now:

1. Make-up ☐
2. Groomed hair ☐
3. Glasses including shades (2 stars for supersized shades) ☐
4. Each piece of jewellery, e.g. watch, different rings, necklace, pair of earrings ☐
5. Contrasting buttons ☐
6. Wearing multi-colours ☐
7. Scarf ☐
8. Belt ☐
9. Patterned/coloured tights ☐
10. Detail on shoes (e.g. sling back, peep toe) ☐
11. Nail polish (1 star for subtle, 2 stars for bright colours) ☐
12. Handbag ☐

---

10 stars are about right for a well-accessorised, dressed up look.

Petite or slightly built? 10 is the maximum. Tall women can carry off up to 13.

If you're struggling to tick 5, take care you don't look a 'plain Jane'.

Over 14? Less really is more – save that diamante choker for tomorrow.

KEEPING CURRENT

Style sense

So why do accessories matter so much? Can you think of a better way to update your look for less than a tenner? What about making a statement – how else can you so easily say who you are? What do your Burberry bag or your Prada shoes say about you? What about that bracelet everyone compliments you on? No-one would know, or care, that it came from Oxfam. Or that fantastic beaded bag from Butler and Wilson which makes you feel so special?

Accessories draw attention so you can use them as a distraction tactic. There's no better way to take attention away from gargantuan thighs or mega butts than drawing the eye elsewhere, perhaps to your fantastic décolletage enhanced by the latest necklace. Fantastic hands and a manicure to die for? Don't waste it; turn them into eye candy by wearing rings, a watch or bracelet. Slim, sexy ankles? The right shoes will show them off beautifully.

You may read this and think it doesn't apply to you. You've never been an accessories girl – one rucksack and a pair of trainers is all you need. Perhaps so, but don't stop reading yet as with just a little time, a few pounds, and a creative imagination you'll be amazed at the difference the right accessories can make.

'Having very short hair I ALWAYS wear earrings & eyeliner, it reinforces my femininity (to me at least).' Anonymous

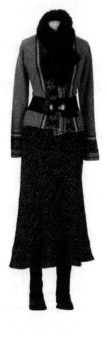

Activity
Jazz it up

- Take an outfit of yours which you like but needs a bit more oomph. Lay it out and decide which types of accessories would make a real difference. Either use ones you already possess or look through magazines and catalogues to get some ideas.

- Take a trip into town and see if you can buy one or two adornments to create the look you want. Do this on a budget of less than £50.

KEEPING CURRENT

159

Scent of a woman

Smell: the most basic and probably the most underused of our senses. Like a signature handbag, perfume is the ultimate luxury accessory that can convey instantly who you really are.

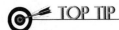

TOP TIP

◆ Never test more than three fragrances at once because your nose will become confused.

To many women, choosing a perfume is a bit like ordering wine in a restaurant – completely terrifying. As Griselda stares at you from behind the counter, fiercely guarding her sample bottles, panic sets in because you don't know where to start. Well, here are some pointers.

For a start, never buy a perfume because it smells good on your friend. You will know that some are, well, hideous, and others are absolutely stunning. The thing about perfume is that it's designed to react to your skin, so it will smell differently on every woman. Try it before you buy it.

Perfume smells are called notes. Although perfumers all have their own definitions, the average nose can distinguish between two main types of notes: oriental and floral. Every perfume has a unique blend of different notes mixed together so you can choose one that appeals to your mood, personality and the occasion.

Oriental notes are heady and heavy, and are made from ingredients such as vanilla, cumin, sandalwood, musk, cinnamon and nutmeg. Perfumes with lots of oriental notes include Chloe Collection 2005.

Floral notes are light and fresh and made from ingredients such as jasmine, lemon, rose, peony and tuberose. Joy by Jean Patou is a great example of a classic floral fragrance.

Perfume also comes in different concentrations that will set you back varying amounts. Eau de Toilette is the cheapest and most diluted. It's often a spray and you can use it every day for work or after sport. Parfum (perfume) is never a spray and will cost the most because it's the most concentrated. Eau de Parfum is more concentrated than Eau de Toilette and less than Parfum and costs somewhere in between.

Activity

Sniff test

- Go to the perfume counter in your local department store. Pick up a perfume you already know and like.

- Spray it on your wrist and smell it immediately

- Spray it in the air and leave it for a moment before walking into the mist. Smell it now – the scent will have opened up and it will be more full and delicate.

- Finally, spray a blotter paper and smell it immediately. Leave it a few moments and smell it again.

- Notice how all of these methods will give you different strengths of smell. Next time you choose a new perfume, make sure you do the full sniff test before you buy.

KEEPING CURRENT

Personality pick

It's helpful to know who makes accessories that match your personal style. Here are a few of our favourites. Some are high street names, others are designers and several you'll only find on the internet.

Simply stylish – elegant and understated. Be subtle and coordinated. Choose great quality. Make sure you keep up to date and avoid looking mumsy.

Designer	High street	Online
Hermes	Jane Shilton	cabouchon.com
Aquascutum	Radley	linksoflondon.com
Chanel	Fendi	icecool.co.uk
Furla	Ralph Lauren Polo	net-a-porter.com
Burberry	Coccinelle	
Orla Kiely	M&S Autograph	
Philip Treacy	Gabor	
Wright and Teague	LK Bennett	
Prada	Georg Jensen	
Jimmy Choo	Next	
	Phase Eight	

Drama queen – trendsetting and noticed. Choose striking, bold, large designs for impact. Use focal points. Do you know how to do discreet?

Designer	High street	Online
Philip Treacy	Karen Millen	ebay.co.uk
Stephen Jones	TopShop	agentprovocateur.com
Luella	Pied À Terre	asos.com
Moschino Cheap and Chic	Nine West	net-a-porter.com
Pucci		accessorieslounge.com
Manolo Blahnik		blissfulbags.com
Versace		
Jimmy Choo		

KEEPING CURRENT

Au naturel – Practical and unfussy. Choose natural materials and simplicity. A selection of interesting accessories will enhance your look in seconds. Beware of looking drab.

Designer	High street	Online
Mulberry	Gap	boden.co.uk
Stella McCartney	Birkenstock	net-a-porter.com
Emporio Armani	Hogan	toastbypost.com
Anya Hindmarsh	Kipper	
Miu Miu	Kangol	
J&M Davidson	Olsen	
	Dune	
	Sole Sister	
	River Island	
	Phase Eight	
	Jones the Bootmaker	

Creative chick – You enjoy all sorts of accessories, from vintage to ethnic. Experiment but don't overdo it.

Designer	High street	Online
Stephen Jones	Johnny Loves Rosie	pirateverte.com
Stella McCartney	Jesire	asinnovations.co.uk
Marni	Oasis	ebay.co.uk
Missoni	Accessorize	net-a-porter.com
Marc Jacobs	Monsoon	toastbypost.co.uk
Liberty	LK Bennett	blissfulbags.co.uk
Patrick Cox	Kurt Geiger	
	Butler & Wilson	
	Fenwick	
	East	
	Bertie	

Activity

Take your pick

- Today will help you locate accessories to suit your personal style. Looking for inspiration? This will give you a great start – look through magazines or on websites for ideas. Even better – visit the shops. Add other favourites to the list.

KEEPING CURRENT

Common questions

In case you still have some burning questions around buying and wearing accessories, we've listed some frequently asked questions and answers for you.

Q Must my bag and shoes always match?

A *It's your choice, although precise matching can look more up to date (and gives you many more options).*

Q I have feet which are a size 8, and I'd rather they didn't look any bigger. Any advice?

A *Go for shoes with a bar or strap across the foot, or any type of horizontal design detail. Avoid pointed toes as these will lengthen your feet unnecessarily.*

Q I'd love to wear boots but can't get them to fit my calves.

A *Try Duo of Bath (duoofbath.co.uk) who have a great selection of different width fittings on boots.*

Q I have warm colouring, but I dislike yellow gold. What jewellery can I wear?

A *Try silver with colours such as amber, jade or malachite, or fantastic ethnic beads, coral, wooden or copper pieces to really complement your colouring.*

Q My neck has gone turkey-like, so I don't like showing off my décolletage any more. However I also have a large bosom and so can't wear high necks. Any advice?

A *Try a slightly higher neckline (but not polo or cowl) and then accessorise with a great pendant to create a 'pseudo V'. Just ensure this doesn't overhang your bosom. Alternatively, a neat scarf tied into a knot in your neckline can also work well.*

Q **I'm tall and also a size 18/20. What size of accessories will help me to look less gigantesque?**

A *Aim for large accessories as tiny, itsy bitsy ones will make you look bigger in comparison. Go bold and be adventurous – you can wear some really magnificent, eye-catching pieces.*

Q **I'm short and thin. Can I wear a hat?**

A *Yes. But don't go for a large hat – keep it quite delicate like your features. A lighter colour will help you to look taller too.*

Q **I've got really thin ankles – would chunky heels help to make them look less sparrow-like?**

A *No – best to go for slim heels which will show off your delicate ankles. Hefty heels will make them look stick-like.*

Q **I love rings – is it ok to wear them on most fingers?**

A *Best not to – 'ring' the changes each day, rather than wearing them all together, which looks cheap.*

Q **My neck's quite short – is it OK to wear chokers?**

A *Afraid not – chokers will visually shorten your neck, as will dangly earrings. Try pendants or beads instead.*

Activity

Any questions?

- Think about how you use accessories and any further questions you may have. If you have any questions, type them into ask.co.uk, and see what answer you get. If that doesn't help, seek the help of a pro.

KEEPING CURRENT

Your notes

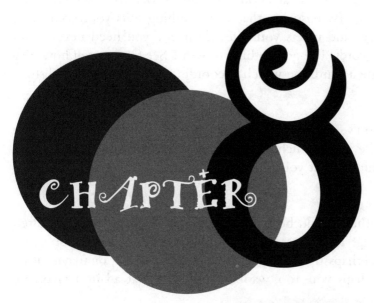

CHAPTER 8

**WARDROBE
WISDOM**

Clobber check

What costs you money, causes you problems and often lets you down? All sorts of things spring to mind, but in this case it's your wardrobe.

'Wardrobe wisdom' is all about creating a wardrobe which really works for you. By ensuring that your clothing suits your colouring, shape, budget and meets your lifestyle needs, you need never again utter those words, 'I've got nothing to wear!' See for yourself how easy it is to create a wardrobe which is coordinated, flexible and stylish.

It's likely you've got many items which you hardly wear, as well as a few favourite items which you wear most of the time. Why does this happen? Think about your shopping habits …

Buying clothes should be a pleasure; however, many of us do often get it wrong. There is so much choice, we buy items for many reasons – perhaps the advice of a friend or partner, or maybe it's a bargain. Perhaps you, too, want to look like that ad in a favourite magazine?

> **FACT**: Most women wear just 20% of their clothes 80% of the time.

 TOP TIP

- If you are tempted to buy something, check out whether it will go with at least three items you already posses. If not, be strong – put it back as you may never wear it.

WARDROBE WISDOM

Activity

Look lively

- Take a look inside your wardrobe. Answer the following, honestly:

  1. How many clothes were **not** worn in the last year?

  2. How many of your clothes are worn regularly?

  3. How easy is it to see which clothes you've got?

  4. Do you feel excited (or depressed) when you open the wardrobe door?

- Now, decide if your wardrobe needs some TLC!

- In your notebook list down why you sometimes buy things which, frankly, never see the light of day.

WARDROBE WISDOM

Declutter

It's time to be ruthless. Now that you've looked at your wardrobe and estimated how much you own which you don't wear, you need to take action. If you haven't worn a garment for over a year you're very unlikely to wear it in the future (even if it did cost a

FACT Recent studies suggest on average, women waste around £500 a year on clothes they don't wear.

month's salary). The only exception to this are special occasion clothes, or if you've had a major life change such as pregnancy. Even if you've lost or gained weight and therefore your clothes don't fit, you're unlikely to want to wear them in the future if your weight changes.

By clearing out your wardrobe you'll feel like a new person. You'll be able to see what you've got, find clothes quickly, your clothes will hang better and last longer and you'll be able to see where the gaps are in your wardrobe.

 TOP TIP

◆ If you can't bear to chuck a well-loved garment, but you no longer wear it – don't put it back into your wardrobe. Put it in a suitcae or storage box for six months. **If you don't miss it or wear it over that time, then get rid!**

WARDROBE WISDOM

Activity

Clear out your closet

● Take **all** of your clothes out of your wardrobe –
  include underwear, footwear etc.

● Sort them into three piles – **keep, bin, needs
  attention**. To help with this, ask yourself:

  1. Does it suit me?

  2. Do I feel like a Diva when I wear it?

  3. Did this go out with Duran Duran?

  4. Have I actually worn it in the last 12 months?

  5. Does it go with anything else?

  6. Does it suit my lifestyle?

  7. Am I hanging onto the memory or the item
     itself?

● Take the **bin** pile to a charity shop, give clothes
  to a friend or sell them at a dress agency.

● For the **needs attention** pile – take action within
  two weeks. (Otherwise they go!)

● The **keep** pile has clothes which fit and which
  you **have actually worn** in the last year, they
  suit you and your lifestyle. They make you look
  good and feel great. The only clothes you should
  keep that you've not worn in the last year are
  special occasion wear like evening gowns,
  funeral wear, etc. Even then they should go if
  they're over five years old. Make sure these are
  clean and ironed before you get organised.

WARDROBE WISDOM

Optimum organisation

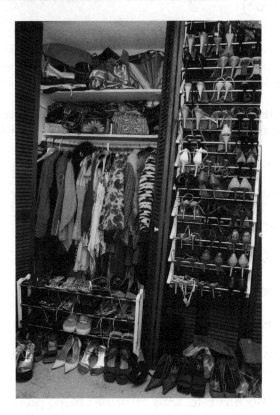

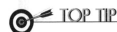 TOP TIP

♦ Avoid wearing the same suit for two days running and always let suits and jackets air for some time after wearing.
♦ If you stain a favourite garment – act fast! Rinse egg, blood, alchol, fruit, tomato and grass stains in cold water only, to avoid 'setting' them.
♦ Need a shirt or blouse quickly? Hang it in the bathroom or dampen in the drier with a damp towel. Iron the sleeves, cuffs and down the middle – the rest will be tucked in.
♦ Add fabric softener to reduce that saucy static.

WARDROBE WISDOM

Activity

Your 7 steps to wardrobe bliss

1. Repair, alter, clean and restore. Deal with your 'needs attention' pile.

2. Make space. Divide by seasons. Store seasonal clothes in airtight boxes or bags and pack them away. Ensure you can see everything you have left and can get at what you need without having to rummage.

3. Get hanging. Don't cram. Double hanging is a good way to make the most of space to accommodate more clothing – ideal for jackets, shirts, skirts and shorter items. Arrange clothes by type, for example blouses, and then by colour tone. Separate suits so you can mix and match at your leisure. Never use wire hangers and get rid of dry cleaning bags.

4. Fold items and smalls. Line drawers with paper or use dividers to ensure everything stays upright, tidy and in place. Stack T shirts, sweaters and jerseys in low piles for good visibility and easy access.

5. Display accessories. Use over-door pockets, tie racks, rails and pin boards on the inside of your cupboard so you can see at a glance what you have.

6. Sort your shoes. Use the floor of your wardrobe for shoes you wear on a regular basis. Pair them heel to toe to maximise space. Put shoes you don't wear often in colourful windowed boxes, or stick a photo of the shoes on the front.

7. Audit and plan. Now you've decided what to get rid of and can see what you want to keep, it's time to take stock of what's left, make some new exciting outfit combinations, and make a plan to fill any gaps.

WARDROBE WISDOM

Accessory audit

The same degree of orderliness should also apply to your accessories. Change your accessories every day to complement your 'look'. If it's like searching for a needle in a haystack it just won't happen. Let's make it happen!

First thing, sort out your crud. Do you wear that necklace that you bought from the little girl with the big eyes in Egypt? If not, surely it needs to go? For unwanted accessories you can give them to a friend, sell them through ebay, or take them to an agency.

Jewellery junk

This is the time where you get rid of any jewellery which is:

◆ Never worn (unless it's your inheritance)
◆ Broken (and not worth repairing)
◆ More dated than designer
◆ Not right for you – the wrong size or style.

Bye bye bags

Maybe you can't imagine ditching a bag until it's beyond tatty and ready to be replaced? If you've got bags which are never used or just plain 'last century', then it's time to get tough.

Shoe shake up

The same rules apply – shine or shove.

Sensible storage

You may have already started this – now you know what to keep and what to clear from your accessories, there are no excuses left. The golden rules for storing accessories are **accessibility** and **visibility**. Stuff hidden under mounds of other stuff will not be worn.

◆ Ideally, store shoes in boxes (with a photo on the front) or on racks or shoe rack cupboards. Use shoe trees where possible.
◆ Any hats should be in hat boxes, wrapped in tissue paper.
◆ Hang belts, scarves and even necklaces and bracelets inside cupboard doors or on hooks so you can see them.
◆ Earring caddies are great, or you can pop them in a well ordered jewellery box.

TOP TIP

◆ Ikea and Lakeland have some great storage solutions. Look on the internet for inspiration.

Activity Accessory audit

● Give your accessories a clean-out. Look for storage systems which work for you.

WARDROBE WISDOM

Time twister

As you clear the clutter of your wardrobe you need to think about your lifestyle. This is really important in getting the balance of clothes right within your wardrobe – there's no point in having six ball gowns if your name's Avril Lavigne.

To help you do this in more detail, think about your typical day.

How do you spend your time? Think about your work, your family activities, any housework. What about hobbies – going to the gym or watching TV? Be honest with yourself. Are you a couch potato or marathon mad?

Now you've done that, what about things you do on a weekly basis – visiting others, entertaining, going out, clubbing?

Don't forget annual events. Maybe this includes going to the gym (in which case no need to spend a fortune on the latest gym gear). What about holidays, annual balls, conferences? If your only social event is on New Year's Eve, don't kid yourself that those eight evening bags are going to wear out …

WARDROBE WISDOM

Activity

Happy hour

- The average person spends 10 hours per day sleeping, getting ready for bed, getting up and eating. That leaves 14 hours per day or 98 hours per week. What do you do in your 98 hours?

- In your notebook, draw a graph with hours per week along the left and different activities you do along the bottom. Then work out approximately how many hours per week you spend on average on each activity and plot it as a graph. It should look a bit like this:

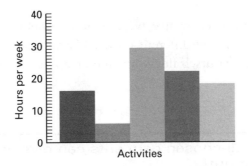

For example, if you estimate that of your available time of 98 hours you spend 40 hours working, this is the amount you will shade in your graph.

- Jot down the types of clothes you need for each activity – how much formal business wear, or 'smart casual'?

- Of course this exercise may bring to light more than the types of clothes you need, it may force you to consider your lifestyle itself.

WARDROBE WISDOM

Creative capsules

Think back to yesterday's activity when you faced some home truths about your lifestyle and where you spend most of your time. Today you are going to pull it all together into a wardrobe full of clothes which you love, are flexible and which reflect the real you.

Take a look at your wonderfully sorted wardrobe – wow – bet it looks great. Now, bearing in mind the analysis you've already done, how does the content of your wardrobe stack up? Do you have enough of the right garments, or are you facing a wardrobe with more gaps than a toothless smile?

No worries – time to plan your investment.

Capsules are not rocket science, but a small set of clothes which work together to make many different outfits. Capsules are a brilliant and cheap way to give yourself flexibility and creativity with your clothes.

Capsule keys

> **FACT**: 12 well-chosen garments can give you up to 88 different outfits.

Colour You will know your best 'neutrals' from Chapter 3. These are the foundation to your capsule – they work brilliantly for suits, jackets, skirts, trousers, coats and accessories. A well-chosen neutral will give you loads of options for other 'accent' colours. For instance, if navy is your chosen neutral, you could choose pink, red, turquoise, white, cream or lilac to go with it.

Balance Always follow the 80/20 rule for maximum flex. This means, within a capsule, choose 80% of clothes for your top half and 20% for your lower half. See opposite for an example of this.

WARDROBE WISDOM

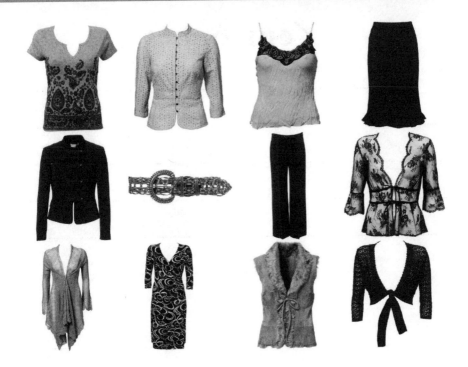

Activity
Your capsule

- Look at the capsule above as an example. In your notebook list items which you could put into your capsule. Either base it around garments you already possess, or build it from scratch.

- If you feel stuck for inspiration, create a montage of pictures from catalogues or magazines to give you some ideas.

WARDROBE WISDOM

Your notes

CHAPTER 9

SHOPPING SURVIVAL

Shopping sherpa or retail recluse?

How many times have you been shopping for clothes and returned home with nothing at all, or worse still with armfuls of impulse buys that you've worn once and then pushed to the back of the wardrobe? Now you know what suits you, it's time to look at what's missing from your current wardrobe and hit the shops to fill some gaps.

Someone once said their relationship with shopping was as complex as the one they had with their mother. If you can relate to that, you're in need of help. Whether you usually hit the high street or prefer to order clothes by mail order from the comfort of your sofa, over the next few days, you're going to learn how to buy only items that really suit you, how to get value for money from your purchases and how to stay sane in the process.

Try out this quiz. See how you score.

Activity

Shopping quiz

1. Does the idea of shopping fill you with dread?
2. Do you return from the shops with armfuls of stuff but still have nothing to wear?
3. Have you been visiting the same shops for more than five years?
4. Is there any item of clothing (apart from your wedding dress) that you have only worn once in the last year?
5. Do shop assistants sneer at you?

Give yourself 1 point for each 'yes' answer. Add together the number of points here: _____

SHOPPING SURVIVAL

6. Can you name three items that will update your look this season?

7. Do you have a list of favourite shops that usually stock styles and sizes to suit you?

8. Do you have a trusted alterations person?

9. Do you know the item of clothing in your wardrobe with the lowest cost per wear?

10. Do you know which shops provide free personal shopping services?

Give yourself 1 point for each 'no' answer. Add together the number of points here: _____

Total score _____

7 or more: You avoid shopping where possible, you waste money and you could look better. Get help.

4–6: You have an eye for a bargain, but you sometimes come home with ridiculous impulse buys. You may be stuck in a rut and could learn how to shop more effectively.

1–3: You've got it sorted. Your shopping muscles may benefit from a little toning, and maybe you could improve on your shopping Return on Investment.

SHOPPING SURVIVAL

Your shopping calendar

Do you wait until July to buy a swimming costume, or look for a New Year's Eve outfit during the Christmas holidays, only to find they've sold out or there's nothing in your size? The hard retail truth is that if you wait until you need it, chances are it will be gone. In a bid to boost sales, shops stock garments up to 4 months ahead of the time when you're going to need them!

You have to train yourself to think a season ahead. It's like gardening – if you want lettuces in the summer, you have to plant them in the spring. Here are some shopping calendar guidelines.

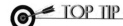
TOP TIP

♦ Get on the mailing lists for your favourite shops so that you receive invitations to sales previews and special events.

December/January: The sales start as early as the second week in December now. Time to buy cut-priced cashmere. If you are prepared to fight the crowds, you can pick up some bargains.

February/March: Spring fashions start pouring in using this season's colours. Fashions go mad for Valentine's Day. This is a good time to buy summer knitwear.

April/May: Serious summer clothes start arriving whilst we're all taken aback by late frosts. Navy shows up and spring clothes go on sale. Buy your swimming costume now.

June: Summer sales start. If you haven't bought summer gear yet, run fast.

SHOPPING SURVIVAL

July: The shops are filled with late summer bargains (or tat) and autumn gear starts appearing. A good time to buy knitwear. Not a swimming costume in sight!

August/September: If you have children, rush to buy their winter uniform before the start of school. This is a great time for autumn knitwear and winter tights.

October: Winter fashions fill the aisles. Clothes start appearing now for the festive season. Time to hunt for your Christmas and New Year season outfits. Stock up on ski-wear now.

November: Resort wear appears now, but for us stay-at-homes this is a dull month for shopping. Exciting clothes are being pushed off the floor by Rudolf and Santa, festive pullovers and furry slippers!

Activity

Your shopping calendar

- List any special events coming up this year that you will need to go shopping for – weddings, social functions, interviews, start of school year, etc. Using the guidelines above, make a note in your diary when you need to shop for them.

- Phone up your favourite shops and find out when their sales start. Make a note of these in your diary too.

- Make sure you put your name on the mailing lists of your favourite shops.

SHOPPING SURVIVAL

Plan of action

These wise words apply to shopping too. Not having a plan is a sure way to return home with nothing, or worse still, armfuls of useless and unsuitable gear you will have to return, or which will fester for years unworn in your wardrobe.

If you're financially solvent to the max, planning and budgeting isn't of great concern: you can afford to buy a completely new wardrobe each season. But for most of us, great shopping starts with knowing what you already have and figuring out what you need to add.

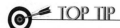 **TOP TIP**

♦ When making your list, don't forget to include underwear. A great outfit can be ruined by the wrong cut or colour underwear. Make sure yours is up to the job.

It's a fact that women who dress with stylish ease build wardrobes around core items such as a trouser suit or jeans, which will last several seasons. They update their look each season with new items, accessories, jewellery, and hosiery. It goes without saying that these suit their colouring, shape, personality and, lifestyle – and, of course, their budget!

SHOPPING SURVIVAL

Activity

Your shopping plan

- Open up your wardrobe, and with the coming season in mind, note down in the first column what you have and its colour.

- Now note down for each item what you already have to go with it. Notice where the gaps are, and where you have items you love, but nothing to wear them with.

- Use fashion magazines such as *InStyle*, *Eve* or *Marie Claire* to pick out at least three new items that will bring your wardrobe up to date. List the items you need to buy to go with what you already have. If you can, prioritise and set yourself a budget. Remember to take your list shopping.

Garment	Have to go with it	Need to buy
Tops		
Bottoms		
Jackets and coats		
Dresses		
Jewellery		
Accessories (shoes, bags, hats, scarves, tights)		

SHOPPING SURVIVAL

Your personal shopping destinations

Knowing what you want to buy is one thing, but do you know where to go for it? High street stores can be so samey, and if you're looking for something a little different, it's well worth doing some research.

There are some great guides available, such as the City Life shopping guide to Manchester. Check out your local information centre or book store to see what's available in your town. It's also worth asking well-heeled friends where they shop – keep a list of boutiques you'd like to visit.

Vintage shopping is also a very exciting opportunity to find unusual buys, but beware – some shops sell vintage ranges that are in the style of older clothes, but in fact brand new. Also, make sure you don't compromise on quality. The definition of vintage seems to vary from shop to shop – in some cases it simply means over 18 months old.

Finally, for armchair shoppers, there are some great clothes and accessories available now online and through mail order catalogues.

Activity

Plan where to shop

Before you spend any money, it's worthwhile considering where you're going to shop. If you always go to the same place, it's probably time for a change. Start this activity by listing where you usually shop, and then add a few new places to your list.

1. High street stores

2. Boutiques

3. Vintage

4. Online / mail order

SHOPPING SURVIVAL

Clothes cost per wear

Have you heard of shopping maths? Good shopping maths isn't just about sticking to a budget – it's also about getting value for money.

For example, a £200 pair of black trousers can seem expensive until you calculate the CPW (cost per wear). Good black trousers are an essential basic in any woman's wardrobe, and a pair that will last more than a couple of years are going to cost less than £1 per outing (OK, excluding dry-cleaning) and are therefore a bargain.

So next time you go out shopping, instead of balking at the price tag, consider instead the cost per wear you're likely to achieve. Perhaps that £50 bargain jacket that you'll only wear twice isn't such a good buy after all.

Here's how to work it out:

$$\text{CPW} = \frac{\text{Cost of item} + \text{cost of cleaning}}{\text{Times worn per week} \times 52 \times \text{no. of years you keep it}}$$

> **FACT**: The average British woman only buys five pairs of pants per year – fewer than any other item of clothing. If she keeps them for two years that works out at less than $1/2$p per wear!

Activity

Do your fashion maths

- Look inside your wardrobe. Pull out the five most expensive items.

- Work out the CPW for each item and compare the results for each.

- Which has been the greatest value for money over the past year?

- Now compare how you feel about each item.

- Next time you go out shopping, do a quick CPW comparison. Is the item you're considering buying worth it in the long run? Could you afford to spend more on this item, even if it means blowing your budget?

SHOPPING SURVIVAL

Ready, steady, shop

Now you're ready to hit the shops. Here are our tips.

Dos

- Ditch the coat. Wear as few clothes as possible so you're comfortable and can easily get dressed and undressed.
- Wear underwear you're proud to be seen in. If possible wear a smooth line, flesh coloured bra – it's the most versatile for trying on clothes.
- Take a bottle of water.
- Wear comfortable shoes that go with skirts and trousers, which you can kick off easily and can walk about in all day.
- Take a pair of evening or high heeled shoes if you're looking for clothes that will need them.
- Wear a bag that hangs across your body so you have both hands free.
- Take your list, your colour swatch and your style 'rules' so you know what to go for and what to avoid.
- Have an idea of the shops you want to visit. If you're using a personal shopper, book ahead.
- Wear flesh-toned tights or bare legs under trousers.
- Take some fresh wipes and deodorant in case you start to melt!

'Behind every shopping woman lurks a kill-joy male and he'll most often say you look fine in something – either to get out of the shop fast or to stay on friendly terms with you.'
Anonymous

Don'ts

Do not:

◆ Wear a thong unless you've got a J-Lo bottom

◆ Shop if you're already tired

◆ Try on trousers with flat shoes if you usually wear them with heels – they'll end up too short

◆ Wear a heavy coat – you'll get hot and end up having to carry it

◆ Take your mum, your man or your best friend unless they can be totally honest or have a very large wallet

◆ Wear tons of jewellery – keep it simple, if you wear anything at all

◆ Have your hair done specially – chances are your style will be ruined by all the trying on

◆ Wear pop socks – they look dreadful with skirts and leave marks halfway up your calves when you take them off

Activity

Get ready to shop

● Use the points above as a checklist to make sure you're in tip-top form and fully equipped for the task ahead.

● See if you can come up with some additional tips of your own.

SHOPPING SURVIVAL

A winner's mindset

You're ready to hit the shops. Your budget's set, you're armed with a list of priority items, you know where you want to go – and suddenly you're overcome with a sense of foreboding. How will you make this trip different from all the others? What can you do to maximise your chances of success?

OK, it's only a shopping trip, let's get a grip now. Everyone goes shopping, don't they?

> **FACT:** Half of all women don't try things on before they buy. Sometimes around three quarters of what they buy goes back.

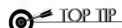 **TOP TIP**

- ◆ If you really hate shopping, get someone else to do it for. Use a free personal shopper from a department store, or hire a professional image consultant to help you.

Activity

Set up for success

As you hit the shops, follow these tips to put yourself into the mindset for success.

- Only shop on high-energy days.

- Do your serious shopping on a weekday and avoid the crowds.

- When you walk into a shop, look first for the colours that suit you. That way, you can ignore everything that's unsuitable. Then focus on shape, texture and style.

- Always try a garment on before you buy and sit down in it to test whether it actually fits. Never believe the size label.

- Use the three-way mirrors in the changing room.

- Never buy anything in the wrong colour or shape, and make sure the item you select will go with at least three other items in your wardrobe. If it doesn't, put it back.

- Never compromise on quality. You usually get what you pay for.

- Never buy an item you're unsure about. If in doubt, wait for 24 hours and come back.

- Don't be bullied by ignorant or over-zealous shop assistants. But make friends with assistants who take a genuine interest, and who go out of their way to find things that really suit you.

- Never purchase anything because it looks good on the shop dummy.

SHOPPING SURVIVAL

Swap shop

What if you can't afford to shop? Don't despair – help is at hand. Have you ever tried a clothes swap party? It's a great way to improve your wardrobe, de-clutter your life and recycle.

Simply invite 10-15 friends to gather all the clothes and accessories they no longer wear and bring them to your home. With wine and snacks you have the perfect afternoon of home shopping as guests take a turn in offering an item to the others. There will be lots of laughter at past mistakes, lots of trying on and bargaining if more than one person likes it, and a fashion show at the end.

Pack off all unwanted items to the charity bin. Everyone will come away with some really nice clothes that will be used rather than hidden at the back of wardrobes. Do try it – it's great fun!

Activity

Organise a clothes swap party

● Invite your friends and ask them to invite their friends. About 10–15 people is the goal – aim for all shapes and sizes.

● Set some clear rules. For example, the original cost of the item doesn't matter; all items must be in good condition and clean; clothes, bags, shoes and jewellery are all worth the same.

● If you are hosting the swap at your house, make sure you have at least two full-length mirrors available.

● For those who are shy, make rooms available to dress and undress.

● Clothes swaps can be seasonal, but they don't have to be: the best clothes swaps have clothing for all seasons.

● If two people want the same item, you can have fun with this by either a coin toss, or having each person model the item of clothing and have a vote (do this only if you're sure there won't be hard feelings).

● If you have second thoughts about an item you're offering, speak up quickly. A simple 'Hmm, I'm not so sure I'm ready to give that up yet,' should suffice, before someone else gets too attached to the item.

● Be prepared – for a good time! You'll be surprised how much fun you'll have with a group of women trying on clothing.

SHOPPING SURVIVAL

Are you keeping up? Do you need some help? If you've not already subscribed, why not try the daily text messaging service for extra encouragement and support. Just text 'Fab 91' to 80881 now.

Each set of messages costs £1.50. Please see page xiii for full terms and conditions.

Dressing up time

Play dressing up. Do you remember when you were little – did you have a fashion show once the shopping bags were brought back home? There's something so delightful about sharing with someone else the things you bought on a successful shopping trip. Do you have someone to play dressing up with: a girlfriend, your buddy, a sister, mother, husband, boyfriend, your kids. Share your success with a trusted person who will be happy for you. And if that isn't possible for some reason, get dressed up in one of your new outfits and go to the local supermarket or off to the pub. Feel as pretty as a peacock. You look great!

Finally, ignore your grandmother's advice – don't save your glad rags for best – you'll never wear them. Wear them now!

SHOPPING SURVIVAL

Activity

Have fun with a fashion show

- Unpack all your bags and lay out your purchases on the bed.

- Using your list of items to mix and match, put together two or three outfits with your new purchases.

- Get some wine out, play some music, create an atmosphere.

- Get dressed up, do your make-up, wear your accessories.

- For each outfit, imagine you're someone famous. Get into the groove. What might they say, how would they walk, what would they feel like inside?

- Strut your stuff and see what reaction you get!

- Remember – **you're worth it**.

SHOPPING SURVIVAL

Your notes

CHAPTER 10

HELPING HANDS

Helping hands

By now, you're well on the way to a new, confident you. With any luck, you will have received positive comments and gasps of excitement and delight from your friends as you step out, attractive and glowing.

But what if you still want a little outside help? The next few days are designed to steer you in the right direction and provide you with tips and advice on how to find help and get the most from the people you turn to. You'll be surprised that the best advice doesn't always need to cost a fortune. But if it does, make sure it's worth the investment.

Activity

Do I need a helping hand?

Work through the following test honestly and see if you'd benefit from a little professional advice.

1. I've followed the advice in this book but I am still unsure about what suits me and how to develop my personal style.

   Yes? Seek help from a professional image consultant or stylist.

2. My looks have improved, but I'm still lacking in self-confidence and I need a boost to help me focus and keep me on track.

   Yes? A life coach could give you the support you need and help you regain your sense of inner confidence and self-esteem.

3. I've got some great clothes, but if I'm honest, they don't fit me as well as they should.

   Yes? Find a seamstress or tailor.

4. I can't find what I'm looking for in the shops. I really want to have something made especially for me.

   Yes? A designer or seamstress can make to your specifications.

5. With all I know, I still find shopping a chore. I can't bear communal changing rooms and hate all the traipsing around.

   Yes? Enlist the services of a personal shopper.

6. My body's sorted, but my hair and face still look a mess. I'd really benefit from a spot of grooming.

   Yes? Get yourself to a hairdresser or beautician.

7. I'm happier with my body as it is now, and I know how to dress to make the most of my assets. In fact it's given me the confidence and will power to lose weight and get fitter.

   Yes? Find a dietician and/or a personal trainer who can work with you.

HELPING HANDS

Image consultants and stylists

Image consultant, stylist – what comes to mind is Trinny and Susannah or Carole Caplin, one-time stylist and lifestyle advisor to Cherie Blair. In reality, there's a whole industry of people working quietly behind the scenes to transform you from bag lady to beauty queen.

If you've followed the advice in this book, you may be doing very well already, so why would you call on them? Here are a few reasons.

◆ You want an objective second opinion about how to make the most of your looks and you won't get it from your friends or your mother.
◆ You can't afford to experiment and risk making a poor first impression.
◆ You're short of time and need someone to take you in hand.
◆ You want to take advantage of their local knowledge of shops and boutiques that will stock garments to suit you.
◆ You want to benefit from their creative flair in putting together looks for a new you.
◆ You want to be pampered.

They're all perfectly valid reasons, and sometimes paying a highly skilled and experienced professional is what's needed to help make changes stick. So how do you go about finding one, and what do they cost? There are three main sources you should turn to.

◆ The Federation of Image Consultants (www.tfic.org.uk) can provide you with a list of qualified image consultants in your area.
◆ Look in the Yellow Pages or Thomson directory under 'Image Consultants'.
◆ Friends who look good themselves may be able to recommend someone who has helped them.

As for fees, they vary greatly – from about £125 for a basic colour or style analysis lasting $1^1/_2$ hours, to £500 per day for a complete package including full image consultation, make-up, and wardrobe review. Accompanied shopping usually starts about around £40 per hour. In all cases, you should shop around and check what you're getting for your money.

Activity

Image consultant checklist

- Use the following checklist to help you choose an image consultant or stylist. You should be able to tick at least six out of eight of these. If you can't, look elsewhere.

1. The consultant should ideally have received appropriate training. For image consultants, this may be with a training provider recognised by the Federation of Image Consultants. ☐

2. Can the advisor demonstrate significant on-the-job experience and a track record of successful work with previous clients? ☐

3. Have you seen testimonials from previous clients? ☐

4. Will you 'get on' comfortably with this person? ☐

5. Do they look good themselves, i.e. do they follow their own advice? ☐

6. Has he/she listened to your needs and objectives? ☐

7. Does he/she appear to be up to date with methods, trends and ideas? ☐

8. What learning materials (such as colour swatch booklets, style advice, pictures, displays) are available to support and reinforce learning? ☐

9. Do they offer a range of services – including at least three of: advice on colour, shape, style, wardrobe management, shopping, special occasion dressing? ☐

Adapted from *Your Guide to Image Consultancy* published by First Impressions, www.firstimpressions.uk.com and www.yourguidetoimageconsultancy.co.uk

HELPING HANDS

Instore freebie

Are you one of the many women who simply drag themselves from shop to shop? Perhaps you don't want to pay for help, but you'd still like some creative input about how to put all your good advice into practice.

> **◎⚡ TOP TIP**
>
> ◆ Some (but not all) personal shoppers work on commission. If in doubt, ask. If they are focused on selling, you may not always get the objective advice you want.
> ◆ Book before you go.

If so, there's great news for you. Many high street stores now offer free in-store personal shoppers who can tend to your every whim and need. And you don't have to be an A-list star. TopShop, Selfridges, John Lewis and House of Fraser are just a few but there are many others. You can ring ahead to make an appointment and discuss your needs. Then, in the comfort and safety of your own personal, luxury-sized changing room, you can try on armfuls of outfits brought to you by willing assistants who will ply you with refreshments and snacks.

A good personal shopper will have a strong sense of personal style and will be trained on the shop floor. They will listen carefully to your needs and take into account your style, colouring, shape and budget. They will also know what's in season, what's in stock and what items cost. If you're a regular, they might put stock aside for you.

Activity

Shop with a pro

- Book an afternoon off with a girlfriend and make an appointment with a personal shopper at a local department store.

- Give them a call in advance and describe your needs. You might find it useful to describe to them what you've already learned suits you, and give them the list of clothes you need based on the wardrobe-planning exercise you did earlier.

- Do it, then answer these questions.

  1. Did you have fun?

  2. Did you buy anything? If so, was it an item on your list?

  3. How much pleasure will you get wearing it?

  4. What do you estimate will be the cost per wear of each item?

  5. What did the experience feel like at the time?

  6. Was it enjoyable?

  7. Did you feel in control?

  8. How confident would you feel to do it again?

  9. How has it made you feel about going into a shop unaccompanied and pulling outfits off the rails yourself?

HELPING HANDS

A stitch in time

When a man invests in a new suit and finds it fits in most places but not in a vital few, he won't hesitate to get it altered. If a man has a large bottom and the trouser pockets gape, it's not an issue, it just means the trousers are the wrong shape and need to be let out so his backside can fit in them. It's the trousers that are the problem, not his bottom! And spending an extra £15 is just part of the investment – after all, why pay £200 upwards for a suit that doesn't quite fit when you're going to wear it every other day? Oh, how refreshing and liberating it would be if women could think that way.

So next time you try something on that's the right colour, a great shape, suits your personality, budget and lifestyle, but whose arms come up an inch too short, think like a man – ask to have it altered. And if you have clothes in your wardrobe that need altering, either do it yourself or find a good seamstress. But above all, don't blame your body.

HELPING HANDS

Activity

Find a good seamstress

Use the following checklist to help you find a good seamstress who can do alterations, and possibly also design or make garments from scratch.

● Be aware that most stores and boutiques will offer an alteration service. There is usually a charge for this.

● If you already own the garment, contact your local fabric stores or the place where you bought it. They may have a listing of local seamstresses to recommend. They may also know them personally and be aware of the quality of their work.

● Ask to see samples of the work they have done already. If that's not possible, ask to speak to clients they have previously worked for.

● Ask how much notice they need for alterations.

● Agree up front how much they will charge.

● Once you've decided to hand over your garment, make sure they mark up the alterations whilst you are wearing the item. It's impossible to just guess.

● Only hand over one item at a time. That way, you can go somewhere else if you don't like the result.

HELPING HANDS

Work out, shape up

There are three ways to change the shape of your body: squeeze it in, shape it up, cut it off. If you've tried the first and don't fancy the third, then perhaps you would benefit from the services of a nutritionist or a personal trainer.

TV programmes such as the no-nonsense *You Are What You Eat* have raised the nation's awareness of the importance of diet in our general wellbeing and physical health. Who can forget Dr Gillian McKeith's command to one of her patients to 'diet or die'? If you lack energy, are prone to colds, suffer from IBS or find it hard to maintain your optimum weight, you may benefit from the services of a professional.

Being a nutritionist is still a relatively new arena, so there is no single regulatory body for professionals. We recommend that your first port of call should be your GP – he/she can assess your current health needs and refer you to an expert in your area.

Personal trainers are exactly that – your personal teacher to help you devise and carry out a physical exercise programme to get your body into shape. Some will come to your home and charge upwards of £80 per hour in London, whilst most gyms and health clubs have their own in-house trainers and charge around £40 per hour.

Personal training has seen a real boom in the last 5 years, and as with nutritionists, there is not yet a recognised regulatory body, so don't be afraid to ask about their training. It's important, too, to feel you can trust and get along with this person. As with medicine, personal trainers often specialise, so make sure yours has an area of specialism that suits your particular needs – for example, recovery after illness, building strength or body sculpting.

Remember, though, you'll get the best results if you combine both diet and exercise, so make sure you tell them about each other.

HELPING HANDS

Activity

Do your research

Whether you're looking for help with diet or fitness, it pays to do your homework. Here are a few helpful hints:

- Ask your friends – you'll be surprised how many people have sought help. There's no stigma now. In fact, having a personal trainer or dietician has a certain celebrity kudos!

- Search on the internet. For example, www.handbag.com has lots of information and advice about what to look for in a personal trainer.

- Check out references from past clients. Don't forget to ask what worked less well too.

- Once you've found someone you can work with and trust, give it time and commitment. Don't expect results overnight.

HELPING HANDS

Call a coach

'Physician, heal thyself.' Biblical proverb

If you need help focusing on your image goals, or building your self-esteem, or if you find it difficult to keep on track, you may benefit from the help of a life coach or personal coach.

This fast-growing and incredibly powerful form of personal development can really help you get results. Most forms of development (like this book) tell you what to do. You are like a glass, half-full and waiting to be filled. Coaching, on the other hand, starts from the idea that every individual has within them the resources to find their own solutions to their problems – all you need is the drive and motivation to take action. You are like an acorn, which has the potential to grow into an oak.

Coaching can be incredibly powerful because it can help you find your own solutions to your problems. It can help you accept who you are, and play to your strengths, whilst accepting your weaknesses.

'There are no constraints on the human mind, no walls around the human spirit, no barriers to our progress except those we ourselves erect.' Ronald Reagan, 40th President of the United States

As with many other forms of self-development, this is a relatively new profession. However, in the UK, there are several recognised professional forums which you can turn to, including:

◆ International Coach Federation
◆ Association for Coaching
◆ Chartered Institute of Personnel and Development (CIPD)

As with all individual service providers, check them out first and make sure you know what you're getting for your money. Many coaches will offer a free introductory session.

Activity

Quick quiz: Do I need coaching?

1. Do you feel there's something missing from your life?

2. Does it feel as if your life is out of control?

3. Do you set goals and find it hard to achieve them?

4. Is your self-esteem rock bottom?

5. Do you feel that you're at a crossroads and not sure which way to turn?

6. Does your 'To Do' list just keep getting longer – with you going round in circles?

7. Do you find it hard to make decisions?

8. Are you ready to make an investment in your future?

If you've answered 'Yes' to any of the above questions, then perhaps it's time to consider working with a life coach.

Source: Annabel Sutton – Life Coach.

HELPING HANDS

Your notes

....

....

....

....

....

....

....

....

....

....

....

....

....

....

....

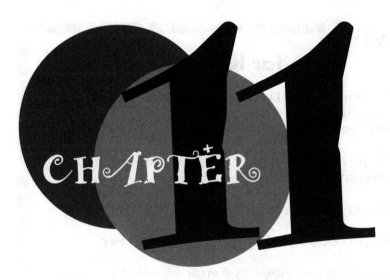

CHAPTER 11

HOW FAR HAVE YOU COME?

How far have you come?

Do you remember at the start of this book, you spent time assessing whether you needed help with your image and self-esteem? Now it's time to see how far you have travelled towards the new you.

Activity

How far have you come?

Take the quiz from Day 2 again and compare the results with those from last time.
Answer 'yes' or 'no' to the following:

1. Do you know what makes you unique and different?

2. Would others say you radiate confidence?

3. Do you buy items to update your look?

4. Do you know how to flatter yourself through choosing the right colours and styles?

5. Do you regularly wear most of what's in your wardrobe?

6. When meeting others for the first time do you generally get a positive reaction?

7. Is clothes shopping enjoyable?

8. Does your make-up look good?

9. Can you list at least five positive things about your image?

10. Can you decide quickly which clothes to wear for most occasions?

How did you do? Score 1 point for each 'yes' and 0 for 'no'.

4 or less: This book will really help you.

5–8: Select your areas of focus – go for it!

8 or more: Great, let's improve on perfection!

In which areas have you made the most progress? Which areas still need some work?

If you still have a low score, try reviewing the chapters that apply to your lowest scoring area and see if there are some additional tips you can pick up.

Confidence A–Z

> 'Self-confidence gives you the freedom to make mistakes and cope with failure without feeling that your world has come to an end or that you are a worthless person.'
> Anonymous

Hopefully you're well on the way to inner confidence, and a new image.

Today is a review of how you can continue to put across your best physical and emotional assets so that the real you shines through.

Activity

Confidence A–Z

- Using your notebook, divide the page into two columns.

- In the left-hand column, write each letter of the alphabet – one letter on each line.

- Now, for each letter, write down one word that describes you at your best or your strongest qualities. These can be inner qualities, such as 'easy-going', or outer qualities, such as 'smile'.

- Once you've done that, use the right-hand column to write down at least one way for each letter that you can let your quality shine through. For example, if you're easy-going, you might choose to wear separates, rather than a suit, to work. Or if you have a great smile, you might choose always to wear lipstick – or brush your teeth more often!

- It may sound silly, but by continuing to take small steps, people will recognise your strengths and qualities, and you in turn will feel better about all the positive compliments you receive. Try it!

HOW FAR HAVE YOU COME?

Goodbye Drab, hello Fab

Congratulations! You've completed 100 steps in the Drab to Fab image and self-esteem personal makeover programme.

How do you feel? Exhausted? Exhilarated? Do you even recognise yourself when you look in the mirror?

Now that you've completed your total image makeover, it's time to take stock of the new you and celebrate your successes.

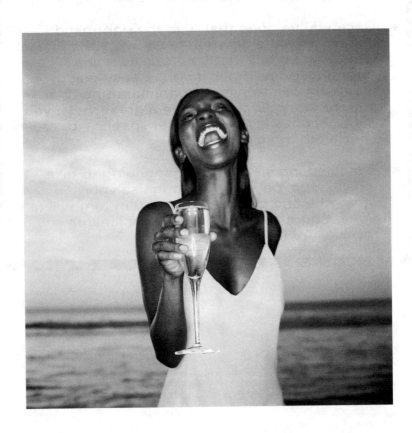

HOW FAR HAVE YOU COME?

Activity

Write your own rule book

- In your notebook, open a fresh page and write in it the top 10 rules you're going to stick to that will help you maintain and improve your new image. Here are some headings to help you on your way.

  - Positive aspects of physical image and personality I want to shine through

  - Three things I will do to create a great first impression

  - Colours that suit me in my wardrobe, make-up, jewellery and accessories

  - Skincare and make-up know-how I will follow

  - Shapes of clothes that work for me

  - Ways I can express my personal style through image

  - Tips to dress for my age

  - Items I promise never to wear or buy again

  - Tips to keeping my wardrobe organised

  - Dos and don'ts to make shopping work for me.

- Take a photo of yourself. Do your hair and make-up and have fun getting dressed up for it. Paste it in your book next to the 'old' you as a reminder of the person you've left behind – forever!

- Ring your friends and arrange a get-together to celebrate the new, improved you. Why not book a pampering treatment for yourselves?

HOW FAR HAVE YOU COME?

Your notes

Your notes

USEFUL CONTACTS

Contact the authors

For advice on how to look good, feel great and raise your self-esteem, contact:

Isabelle Perrett at
iperrett@whattowear.biz and via her website,
www.whattowear.biz

Yvonne Johnson at
Yvonne@create-impact.com

Professional bodies and organisations

The Federation of Image Consultants
www.tfic.org.uk
The Gables, Lammas, Norwich, NR10 5AF
Tel: 0701 0701 018

International Coaching Federation
www.coachfederation.org

Association for Coaching
www.associationforcoaching.com
66 Church Road, London, W7 1LB

Chartered Institute of Personnel and Development
www.cipd.co.uk
151 The Broadway, London, SW19 1JQ
Tel: 020 8612 6200

Toastmasters International
www.toastmasters.org
See website for contact details of local clubs.

Acknowledgements

Our thanks to the following who have kindly given permission to use photos and information for this book:

Hobbs – women's clothing and shoes
www.hobbs.co.uk
Tel: 020 7586 5550

Wallis – women's clothing and accessories
www.wallis-fashion.co.uk
Tel: 0845 1214 520

Figleaves – women's underwear, nightwear and swimwear
www.figleaves.com
Tel: 0870 4999 002

Pirate Verte – women's accessories
www.pirateverte.com
Tel: 0845 0563 782

Stretch Development – David Hyner, professional speaker and trainer
www.stretchdevelopment.co.uk
Tel: 01785 859 589

First Impressions Training – image consultancy training
www.firstimpressions.uk.com
Tel: 01908 393 961

Marks and Spencer plc – high street retailer
www.marksandspencer.com
Tel: 0845 3021 234

Annabel Sutton – Life Coach
www.life-designs.co.uk
annabel@life-designs.co.uk

Kate Everall – photographer
www.kateeverallphotography.com
Tel: 01908 643 767

Francesco Group
www.francescogroup.co.uk

Lewis Moore, Salon Director
Tel: 01785 247175/0121 353 3888

APPENDIX

Women's sizing guide

to fit	size											
	8	10	12	14	16	18	20	22	24	26	28	30
Bust	81 cm (32")	85 cm (33.5")	89 cm (35")	93 cm (36.5")	97 cm (38")	102 cm (40")	107 cm (42")	112 cm (44")	117 cm (46")	123 cm (48.5")	127 cm (50")	132 cm (52")
Waist	64 cm 25"	69 cm 27"	72 cm 28.5"	76 cm 30"	80 cm 31.5"	86 cm 34"	91 cm 36"	98 cm 38.5"	104 cm 41"	109 cm 43"	114 cm 45"	119 cm 47"
Hips	89 cm 35"	93 cm 36.5"	95 cm 37.5"	100 cm 39.5"	104 cm 41"	108 cm 42.5"	113 cm 44.5"	118 cm 46.5"	123 cm 48.5"	127 cm 50"	133 cm 52.5"	138 cm 54.5"

to fit	size					
	8–10 (Small)	12–14 (Medium)	16–18 (Large)	20–22	24–26	28–30
Bust	79–84 cm 31–33"	89–91 cm 35–36"	97–102 cm 38–40"	107–112 cm 42–44"	117–123 cm 46–48.5"	127–132 cm 50–52"
Waist	58–64 cm 23–25"	66–71 cm 26–28"	76–81 cm 30–32"	86–94 cm 34–37"	104–109 cm 41–43"	114–119 cm 45–47"
Hips	86–91 cm 34–36"	94–99 cm 37–39"	104–109 cm 41–43"	112–117 cm 44–46"	123–127 cm 48.5–50"	133–138 cm 52.5–54.5"

Source: Marks and Spencer plc

Why not
try another title in the 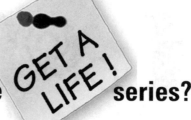 series?

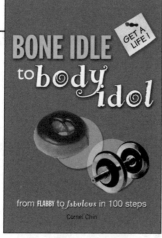

BONE IDLE to BODY IDOL
0-340-90799-1

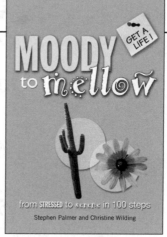

MOODY to MELLOW
0-340-90801-7

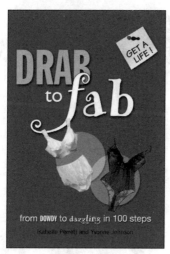

DRAB to FAB
0-340-90804-1

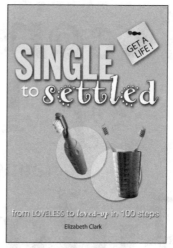

SINGLE to SETTLED
0-340-90800-9

Look Out

for the

GET A LIFE !

Second Wave of Titles

launching in

July 2006

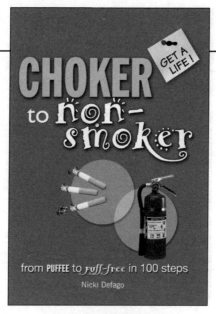

CHOKER to NON-SMOKER

0-340-91540-4

Are you **CHOKING?**
Want to *stop smoking*?
Go from **PUFFEE** to *puff-free* in 100 easy steps!

Top health journalist Nicki Defago will show you how to quit the fags forever and feel great.

How?
Each step of this 100-day program will give you all you need to drop the weed. With 'smoker profiles', interactive quizzes and motivational messages, not only will you give up and stay that way, but you'll also boost your self-esteem. Supporting you at every step, Nicki offers:

* Expert psychological tips
* Self-assessments and daily activities
* Motivational methods
* Strategies for success
* Exercises and emergency plans

Former BBC journalist **NICKI DEFAGO** has written on almost every aspect of women's health for *Eve, She* and *Red.*

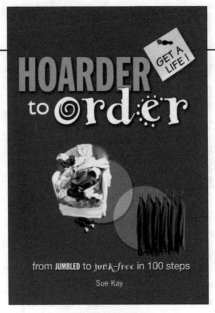

HOARDER to ORDER

0-340-90803-3

Drowning in **JUNK?**
Need to **de-clutter?**

Go from **JUMBLED** to **junk-free** in 100 easy steps!

Decluttering guru Sue Kay is here to help you say goodbye to a muddled head and messy home, and hello to a tranquil and orderly new life!

How?

In just 100 steps you'll go from cluttered to clutter-free, learning habit-changing tips to help you stay this way forever. Don't put it off any longer! Blitz that bedroom and purge that paperwork! This easy-to-follow programme includes:

- ✳ Daily activities
- ✳ Dos and don'ts
- ✳ Action plans
- ✳ Self-assessments and quizzes

Professional Organiser and leading UK declutterer, **SUE KAY's** expertise has featured on the BBC, ITV, and in numerous magazines and newspapers.

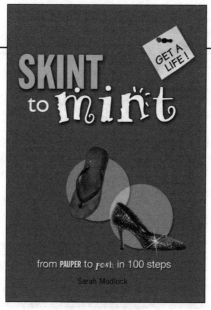

SKINT to MINT

0-340-90802-5

Are you **FINANCIALLY FLABBY?**
Dreaming of a *money makeover*?
Go from **PAUPER** to *posh* in 100 easy steps!

Finance guru Sarah Modlock is here to give you all the advice needed to refresh your bank account, detox your credit card, and achieve lasting financial fitness.

How?

Your 100-step action plan will give you all the advice you need to transform yourself from penniless to plush. From confronting your cash crisis to sensible spending and even saving for that rainy day, your financial freedom beckons. Each step includes:

* Daily activities
* Dos and Don'ts
* Top tips
* Action plans
* Self-assessments and quizzes

You can rely on the expertise of financial journalist **SARAH MODLOCK**, who writes for the major national newspapers and whose articles are featured regularly on Yahoo! and handbag.com.

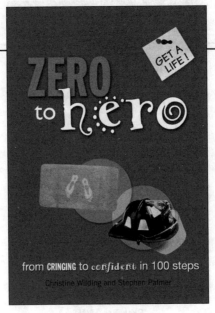

ZERO to HERO

0-340-91539-0

Go from **zero** to h:ero in 100 easy steps!

Professional confidence-boosters Christine Wilding and Stephen Palmer are on hand to help you get perceptive, powerful and positive about every aspect of your personality.

How?

Your 100-step guide to great self-esteem will give you everything you need to cope with a confidence crisis, overhauling your negative thoughts, and turning obstacles into opportunities at work, home and beyond. This practical program includes a toolbox of techniques, tactics, top tips and also features:

* ❊ Daily action plans
* ❊ Questionnaires, quizzes and tick-boxes
* ❊ Motivational stories
* ❊ Ideas and inspiration
* ❊ Key learning points
* ❊ Facts and figures

As a professional behavioural coach **CHRISTINE WILDING** and Founder and Director of the Centre for Stress Management, Professor **STEPHEN PALMER**, are among the UK's most successful confidence coaches.